How to Get Referrals

The Mental Health Professional's Guide to Strategic Marketing

Linda L. Lawless and
G. Jean Wright

John Wiley & Sons, Inc.
New York • Chichester • Weinheim • Brisbane • Singapore • Toronto

This book is printed on acid-free paper. ♾

Published simultaneously in Canada.

Library of Congress Cataloging-in-Publication Data:

Lawless, Linda L.
How to get referrals : the mental health professional's guide to strategic marketing / Linda L. Lawless and G. Jean Wright.
p. cm.
Includes bibliographical references and index.
ISBN 0-471-29791-7 (pbk. : alk. paper)
1. Mental health services—Marketing. 2. Psychiatric referral.
I. Wright, G. Jean. II. Title.
RC465.5.L39 2000
362.2'068'8—dc21 99-23933

10 9 8 7 6 5 4 3

To our colleagues and other professionals who are working hard to survive in the midst of global change, a national reshaping of the healthcare field, and personal and professional challenge.

Preface

Most mental health professionals in private practice are experiencing several challenges in maintaining a vibrant, viable practice. Our primary challenge is related to changes in the traditional referral bases which practitioners have relied on. Our book addresses this challenge and guides you in the building of dynamic referral networks that nurture your practice. We offer tools to help you clarify which marketplace will be the most resonant with your values, skills, and natural gifts.

The book focuses on three primary strands essential to weaving a sustainable practice. First, mental healthcare is local, interacting with and relating to the practitioner's community and region; second, mental healthcare is national, responding to managed care organizations, professional associations, and political, legal, and social issues. Finally, mental healthcare is global, networking with the World Wide Web community and the ecosystemic health challenges of the planet.

While this book focuses on the mental health profession, it also is a resource for anyone working in the healthcare or human service field. Each chapter is a guide that assists you in developing a strategic marketing plan and provides tools for implementation. In all of this, you are the creator and the decision maker.

As we developed this book, we discovered how unique each professional group and their individual situation is. We also found many similarities and the need and potential for us all to work collaboratively to solve local, national, and international problems.

Developing a like-minded peer community quickens the singular journey. We invite you to reach out to us with your insights, successes, and struggles so we can pass this wisdom on to others. The long-term success of your practice requires strategic marketing, patience, tenacity, resilience, and a healthy sense of humor.

LINDA L. LAWLESS AND G. JEAN WRIGHT

Contents

1

Building Blocks for Success

Professional success sometimes comes unexpectedly. More often, it is the result of hard work and perseverance. When your professional goals are congruent with your personal growth path, you will be motivated to work to develop your business. Take the time to evaluate yourself, your life purpose, your professional mission, and your strengths and weaknesses. Use this information to create your personal definition of success and professional goals. William Bridges, in his book *Creating You & Co.* (1997), speaks about the mindset needed to stay viable in a rapidly changing marketplace. Confidence in your abilities is the primary foundation for a successful practice.

Practice development and marketing are necessary activities if you want to achieve success in the mental health marketplace. With more than 395,000 behavioral health professionals in the United States, mental health professionals need to discover new ways to reach the marketplace and provide a return on their investment of time and money (Steenburger, 1997).

With more than 395,000 behavioral health professionals in the United States, mental health professionals need to discover new ways to reach the marketplace and provide a return on their investment of time and money.

The chapters that follow focus on seven professional groups with which you may network to increase your referral base. Beginning with a brief history of a specific market, your awareness of the context of that market increases. Knowledge of your client's historical context can be an essential element in assisting with present issues. Having knowledge of the historical context of the specific marketplace aids you in connecting with and understanding responses to your outreach efforts. Resources are provided for exploring the history of the marketplace you choose.

Getting Started

The work you do requires an awareness of yourself and how you affect your clients. It only makes sense to take who you are into account as you create a professional development plan. Your value system is an important link between you and your professional work. Business values that are congruent with your personal values enhance one another. Some professionals choose to work with a long-term therapy model, while others embrace short-term strategic approaches. Working in a short-term system would create a values conflict for a long-term model therapist.

The value cards in *Organizational Vision, Values, and Mission* (Scott, Jaffe, & Tobe, 1993) are particularly useful. Their system helps you identify your highest to lowest values. Make a list of all your values and then rank them according to priorities. Personal values may include a healthy balance between work, family and friends, loyalty, peace, and so on. Some professional values you may hold in high regard are integrity, client confidentiality, easy availability to patients, and fair compensation for your services. After you have made and ranked your list, compare a value's importance to how saturated your life is with it. When you rate a value highly and are personally dissatisfied with how little you have integrated it into your life, there is a discrepancy that can motivate you as well as guide you in making changes. This book uses an inside-out, organic, approach to practice development. You, your values, and your professional skills become the foundation of your journey to success.

Before you charge down a path toward "success," you must ask what that success means to you.

In *The Wizard of Oz*, as Dorothy and Toto began their journey down the yellow brick road picking up fellow travelers, each character had diverse reasons for setting out on the journey. Each definition of success was vastly different from the others. Before you charge down a path toward "success," you must ask what success means to you. Creating a successful professional practice includes having a clear definition of success, a mission, and a good business and marketing plan. What is a "successful" mental health professional practice? There are many definitions of success. How would you describe the perfect vacation? Each of us might have a different answer, but each could be called successful vacations. We must take responsibility for defining our own success criteria. The average "successful therapist" makes $40,000 to $60,000 a year; the better-than-average therapist may make $140,000 (*Practice Strategies*, December 1997). This data uses income as the primary criteria for the successful therapist. What this doesn't tell us about the therapist is:

- What is that person's quality of life?
- Are the clients interesting?
- Is the work contributing to his or her growth?

These are aspects you should consider when coming up with your own definition of success. Ofer Zur, a psychotherapist and practice consultant in Northern California, identified nine characteristics of a successful therapist in a popular newsletter (*Practice Advisor*, February 1998):

1. Competency.
2. Exploits managed care.
3. Markets to and penetrates managed-care-free markets.
4. Creates self-sustaining referrals.
5. Skilled manager.
6. Develops a special managed-care-free practice.
7. Diversified.
8. Thrives in a practice free of managed care.
9. Avoids burnout.

Zur's perspective of the successful therapist is clearly managed-care-free. However, others' perspectives of success may include group practice issues or managed-care contracts. The definition of a successful mental health professional practice is so wide you must create your own model. No one but you can define your personal model for success.

Once you have defined success, you need to clarify the professional mission that grows out of your life purpose. The mission of your professional practice sets the background for all your goals and plans. It is the big picture that encompasses all your concrete goals and schedules. Examples of a professional mission are:

- To mainstream mental wellness in American culture.
- To remove the stigma from mental illness.
- To create a successful mental health practice in my community that is as healthy for me as it is for my clients.

Because you grow and change as you gain more experience in life, it is important for you to revisit your business mission frequently.

It is vital that you be able to describe your professional practice mission and relate it to who you are. This congruency of how your work grows out of your individual passion is the key to connecting with the clients and customers who can use your services and products.

It is vital that you be able to describe your professional practice mission and relate it to who you are. This congruency of how your work grows out of your individual passion is the key to connecting with the clients and customers who can use your services and products. When you have clarified your values, identified your goals, and created your professional mission, the next step is to design and implement a plan that will help you reach these goals. Now you are ready to begin your journey as a professional/businessperson.

The Mental Health Practitioner as Businessperson

For the mental health practitioner who is in either a solo practice, or in some form of group or partnership, a bottom-line reality is that you also are a businessperson. You are in the business of marketing products and services that facilitate emotional and mental well-being in the community/ies, where your office/s are located.

How to develop an identity as a businessperson is usually not included in the curriculum of professional training programs. Its absence often produces culture shock when the new therapist enters the real world following graduate training. The business side of a private practice creates a learning curve that is often hit or miss. The lack of business skills seriously compromises the potential for a successful professional practice. Our book shows you how to create and implement a strategic marketing/business plan that will grow and nurture your private practice.

If you are already in private practice, you are a self-employed business owner. You are the creator of your practice and are responsible for its viability. The self-employed include a growing number of women. The *New York Times,* Sunday, August 23, 1998, edition, quoting Bureau of Labor Statistics, announced that "of all employed women in 1977, 4.9 percent were self-employed; in 1997, 6.6 percent were self-employed." The Small Business Association reports that women-owned businesses grew 45 percent from 1987 to 1992. If you are a female mental health practitioner in a solo or group private practice, you are most likely part of these statistics. You are a self-employed businessperson and you pay taxes based on that status. *To survive and thrive in the current marketplace, you must integrate this reality—this identity as a businessperson—with your desire to serve and help others.*

An overview of the mental health field conducted by the American Association of Marriage and Family Therapists is a helpful foundation for understanding yourself as a businessperson. In a December 1997 issue of *Practice Strategies,* the organization shared results of their survey of 1,215 private practice therapists. The survey was composed of 55 percent females and 45 percent males and included part-time and full-time private practitioners. A random sample of 457 was carefully composed from the following 5 groups: psychologists (167); professional counselors (104); social workers (75); marriage and family therapists (59); and psychiatrists (52). The practice locations ranged from urban to rural; 68 percent were between the ages of 45 and 65 and had been in practice for an average of 10 to 17 years. Types of private practice were as follows:

- 63 percent of the 1,215 were in a solo practice.
- 18 percent shared space with other solo practitioners.
- 12 percent were part of a professional corporation.
- 1 percent were involved in groups without walls.
- 2 percent were in an independent practice association.
- 4 percent were in a partnership.

For those therapists in full-time practice, the median incomes were:

- Social workers, marriage and family therapists, and professional counselors, $30,000–$39,000.
- Psychologists, $60,000–$69,999.
- Psychiatrists, $120,000–$129,999.

Overhead costs were approximately 25 percent of gross practice incomes. In reporting sources of income, the survey respondents stated that the percentage of their caseload received from managed care ranged from a high of 35 percent to a low of 5 percent. Those in solo practices reported the smallest percentages of caseload derived from managed care organizations. More than half (65 percent–94 percent) of the private practitioner's caseload and income, therefore, must come from other sources. The private practitioner needs to have a diversified

Without managed care referrals, 100% of the income must be generated from other networks.

practice that facilitates the earning of that additional percentage. Without managed care referrals, 100 percent of the income must be generated from other networks.

Your Story

To facilitate your strategic networking with other professional groups, you need to understand factors that affect your self-understanding as a professional. These factors enhance your ability to market your products and services to a diverse community. Tools to aid this process are:

- Your family-of-origin genogram.
- Your therapeutic family-of-origin school.

Your Family-of-Origin Genogram

When you network and connect with other professionals, you first should seek to find those with whom you share common ground and/or areas of like-mindedness. In each of the following chapters, you can use your genogram as a tool to help you choose whether you are interested in developing relationships within that particular group.

It is helpful to first look to your story and your family of origin. A helpful guide in considering the self of the therapist is to work with your family genogram, developed by one of the founding family systems therapists, Murray Bowen, M.D.

If you are unfamiliar with genograms, McGoldrick and Gerson's *Genograms in Family Assessment* (1985) is a useful resource. If you have a computer, software is available for constructing genograms (see Resources). A genogram includes the following three levels (pp. 9–21):

1. *Mapping the family structure.* The genogram, structurally similar to drawing a family tree, is often formulated to show three generations. The three generations to include are your own nuclear family, your parents (family-of-origin), and your grandparents (the third generation). Squares depict males; circles depict females. The identified person (you in this case) is indicated by either a square within a square (if male) or a circle within a circle (if female).

2. *Recording family information*. Family information includes dates of births and deaths, immigrations, marriages, divorces, adoptions, twins, stillbirths, geographic locations, illnesses, addictions, and so on. Putting an "x" through the circle or square depicts deaths. Include date and cause of deaths, if known. Addictions and chronic illnesses are also noted.
3. *Delineating family relationships*. Show who lived with whom; where conflict was in the family; divorces, cutoffs of family members, and so on. The genogram is useful for depicting relationships in remarried families.

We suggest that you focus on a fourth category we feel is essential to greater self-understanding and to relating with other professional groups. This fourth category makes explicit the vocational activities of your family. In this category, include your family members' educational level, work/career categories, and religious traditions.

Also focus on family attitudes about professionals. Family belief systems about such issues are picked up both consciously and unconsciously. These beliefs regarding professionals will be part of your belief system and will affect your responses, your interest or disinterest, your timidity or boldness when marketing your products/services to other professionals. This information is essential to help you understand more about your family-of-origin in the context of its relationship to professional communities.

In addition to a history of work, educational levels, and religious traditions of your family, ask and include in your genogram the following questions:

1. Educational levels:
   - Who first graduated from high school? Dates.
   - From college? Dates.
   - Which college/university?
   - Who first graduated from a graduate and/or specialized training school?
   - How is my education similar and/or differentiated from my family-of-origin?
   - Other questions may arise that are particular to your family.

2. Vocational/work categories:
   - What type of work have/do family members done/do?
   - Who were the first professionals in the family? Which profession/s?
   - How has/does such history impinge on my beliefs/style? My role models are? Why?
   - How is my vocational choice similar and/or different from my family-of-origin?
   - Other.
3. Attitudes:
   - Was the family attitude one of respect and admiration for professionals or was it one of jealousy, anger, apathy, anti-intellectualism?
   - What types of stories were shared, what attitudes were expressed, about professional persons?
   - Was gender a factor in family attitudes?
   - Were my family members engaged in civic activities?
   - Did/do they vote?

Out of the matrix of your family-of-origin experience, what are your beliefs about yourself as a professional and your attitudes about other professionals?

Figure 1.1 shows an example of a simple genogram based on educational, vocational, and religious tradition. Out of the matrix of your family-of-origin experience, what are your beliefs about yourself as a professional and your attitudes about other professionals? Gaining insight and understanding about your personal dynamics, experiences as they relate to your family-of-origin, and your professional life, will help you as you begin networking and communicating with professionals inside and outside the mental health field.

Your story about yourself forms out of this material. Practice telling it as a professional and share it when appropriate as you meet and introduce yourself to other professionals. This information becomes part of the script you develop as a marketing tool. Just as knowing something of the context and characteristics of other professional groups facilitates strategic networking, so having more awareness about your context and family history is an important and helpful element in building bridges of trust to the professional communities you network with.

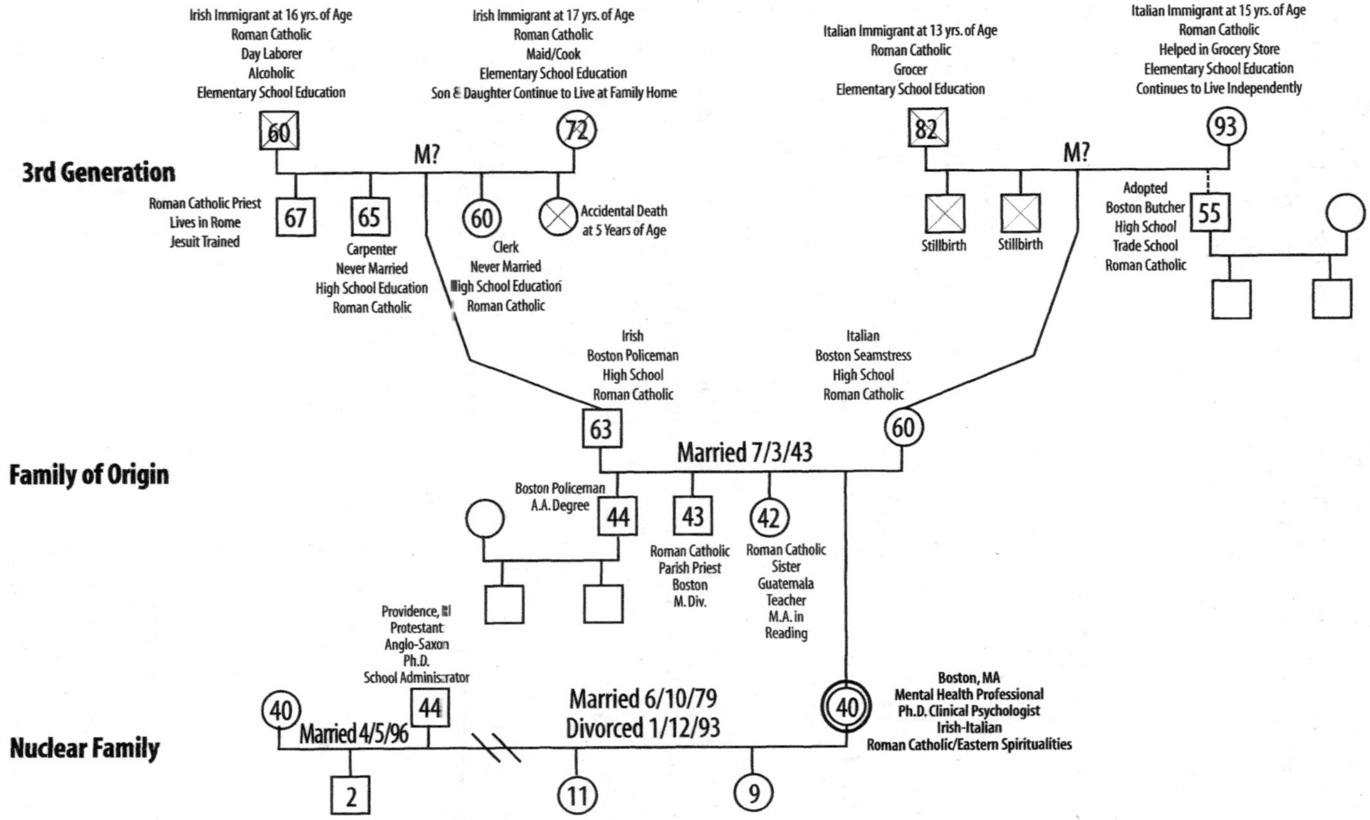

FIGURE 1.1 Sample Genogram of a Mental Health Professional

When you network and connect with other professionals, you should first seek those with whom you share common ground and/or areas of like-mindedness; your family-of-origin story will help you make these identifications. You have clarified an inner standpoint from which to begin the outer work of reaching out and contacting representatives of other professional communities.

Your Therapeutic School "Family-of-Origin"

People have become knowledgeable about schools of psychological thought (due to TV talk shows, movies, and a more educated public) and often ask the mental health practitioner what type of psychology she or he practices. If you apply for acceptance to Managed-Care Organization (MCO) panels, you may have to answer questions about your areas of specialized training and expertise.

Just as developing an understanding of your family-of-origin dynamics regarding your professional life and relationships to other professionals and professional groups adds a critical level of expertise to your marketing ability, so understanding your therapeutic school family-of-origin roots will also empower your professional life.

Understanding your therapeutic school family-of-origin roots will also empower your professional life.

Reflecting on your primary theoretical base for doing therapy, and being able to verbalize it succinctly and clearly enhances your communication about yourself and your practice. Figure 1.2 will assist you in locating yourself in a therapeutic school, and help you develop the information as part of your telephone or written script regarding yourself as a therapist. Practice the script of your therapeutic school family-of-origin several times prior to sharing it with others (see specific chapters for scripts). Tape it, using either audio or video, and listen to your message. Share it with colleagues and ask for their feedback. Develop alternate scripts depending on the group to whom you are marketing.

Visioning and Affirming Your Status as a Businessperson

Create a mosaic of positive images and concepts in your mind to expand the vision and understanding of yourself as a businessperson; a successful civic-minded professional businessperson. The following discussion

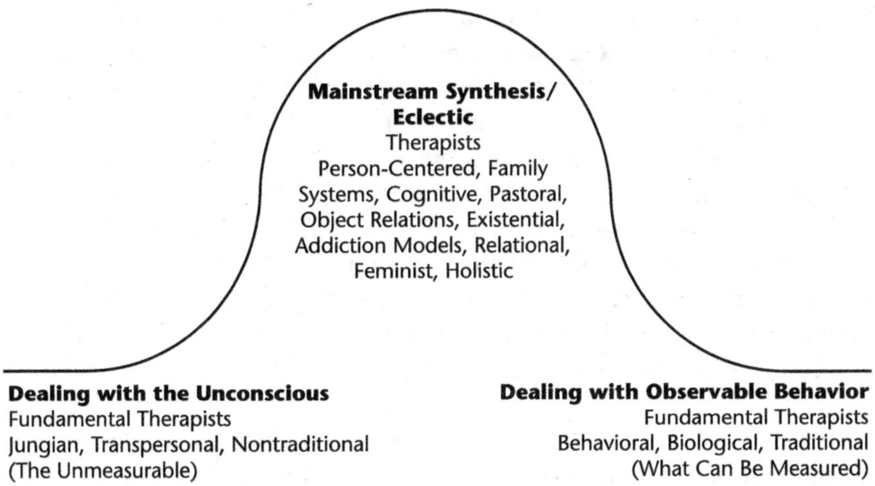

FIGURE 1.2 Locating You and Your "Therapy Family" Tradition

of terms is designed to help you build and envision a successful business in today's market:

Business. A popular definition is employment; occupation; profession; calling; vocation; means of livelihood; that which occupies the time, attention, and labor of men (women), for the purpose of profit or improvement. As a mental health practitioner in private practice, you are in business for both profit and improvement. As you improve the lives of women, men, and children as well as the institutions and communities you touch, you will improve your business outcomes by making a profit.

Altrupreneur. This word is a combination of altruism and entrepreneur. It emphasizes the two realities of private practice mental health professionals: They have chosen the vocation because they love working with and for others and their vocation is a business. Coined by Bernie Nagle and Perry Pascarella (1998), the word means "one who acts with conspicuous regard for the welfare of others" as a first priority and describes leaders who are able to maintain a balance between service and financial responsibility. Private practitioners must have this balance to nurture and promote their altruism and idealism, seasoned with business realities.

Systemic Practice. A basic premise of the ecological and biological world is that environments are connected and sustained within networks of systems and interdependent connectivities. Begin to envision your mental health practice as an entity among other entities of the business community where you work or hope to work and find success. The health and well-being of the community is related to the health and well-being of the businesspeople within it. At the same time, the system is not limited to the local community, particularly in the healthcare field. Due to managed care and the Internet, there is also a national and global system to which the mental health practitioner is related and is a part (whether or not proactively related).

Innovation. Innovative practitioners listen to and receive feedback from the marketplace, attend to the feedback, and design programs, products, and services that are relevant to the market. They attempt various approaches, design systems of accountability regarding the approaches, and let go of what isn't working to test new approaches. They allow death and renewal or extension of products and programs by becoming educated and certified in a particular area of expertise such as eating disorders, attention deficit disorder, or substance abuse. It may also mean reinventing one's niche market. To grow a business, mental health practitioners imaginatively and continually develop new services and products based on the community's needs and their own professional growth.

To grow a business, mental health practitioners imaginatively and continually develop new services and products based on the community's needs and their own professional growth.

An innovative, creative way to develop your marketing plans and service/product design is to use mindmapping techniques. First developed by a teacher, Tony Buzan, to aid student note taking, he soon realized that his construct aided thinking abilities. A book that usefully describes the technique is Joyce Wycoff's (1991) *Mindmapping: Your Personal Guide to Exploring Creativity and Problem Solving* (see Recommended Reading). A software program called "Inspiration" is also available for developing mindmaps (see Resources).

Mindmapping is an important tool that can assist you in creatively developing your strategic plans. Most of the following chapters will make use of the mindmap to begin the strategic networking process to a particular professional group (for an example, see Figures 2.5 and 2.6).

Mindmapping is a creative way to begin brainstorming the constituencies you choose to network with. A mindmap draws on both the right and left sides of the brain and is nonlinear in its development. It is energizing and is an aid to marketing since it allows for movement between the larger picture and the smaller pieces of the plan. The mindmapping tool reduces the feelings of being overwhelmed by the tasks involved in marketing. We have yet to find a problem or issue that cannot be clarified with a mindmap. You can easily construct your own. Make use of color, shapes, forms, and lines to increase your creativity in developing your strategic networking plans.

The mindmap also is a great aid to creativity and organization.

The mindmap also is a great aid to creativity and organization. A basic outline to follow in developing your own mindmap follows. Put the name of the professional group in the center of the page and ask the following questions. (This is a brainstorming activity. Don't allow yourself to get hung up on editing your thoughts. Give yourself 5 to 10 minutes to do this.)

1. *Who.* Who are the groups, subgroups, contacts related to the professional group that I want to target?
2. *What.* What do I want to do in relation to them? What do I need to do based on their needs? What resources do I have available? What resources do I need? What is my budget for this project?
3. *When.* What is my schedule? How long will it take? (The Goal-Setting Worksheet, Figure 2.4, will help answer this question.)
4. *Where?* Where are resources located? Where is the location in which I want it to happen?
5. *Why?* Why do I want to network with this group? Why do I believe I have something to offer them? Why do I believe some of them will respond? Why is it important to me?
6. *How?* How will I measure this strategic networking project? How will I implement it? How will I communicate it? How will I know if it is successful?

By following the mindmapping process, it is possible to have a bare bones plan in 5 to 10 minutes. Play with it! It's fun!

Strategic Networking. Strategic networking recognizes that the wise use of financial resources means focusing your efforts on groups that make a nice fit with your values, mission, purpose, and success goals or can lead you to those individuals. Ivan R. Misner, founder, Business Network International, states: "Networking is a contact sport. . . . Contact with people is the best way to get referrals. You must develop relationships."

Enthusiasm. Mental health practitioners allow their vision for health and well-being to inspire the business side of the practice and can communicate well their reasons for being a business entity in the community. Such enthusiasm is contagious. Review your business mission statement. Practice presenting it prior to strategic networking opportunities. Include it in your brochures, letters, and programs. Allow your enthusiasm to support your business enterprises.

Diversification. Just as having a diversified portfolio in the investment world creates a greater degree of safety and protection for one's financial resources, having a diversified practice and diversified income sources increases the economic base of your practice and income. You need to make the decision about your involvement in the managed-care market as it relates to your income base. Spread referral strategies out among:

- Managed care.
- Self-referrals and self-pay.
- Consultation.
- Teaching.
- Writing.
- Workshop development.

The market is changing so rapidly that it is more useful to think in small increments of time than to develop 5- to 10-year plans.

Sustainability. Develop a sustainable marketing plan for your mental health business that covers 2 to 3 years. The market is changing so rapidly that is more useful to think in small increments of time than to develop 5- to 10-year plans. We suggest a simple design, which focuses your plan on the present as well as the future and maintains a dynamic process between the present and future. The adapted S-shaped sigmoid curve (Blanchard & Waghorn, 1997) depicted in Figure 1.3 is helpful in developing a sustainable market plan. Ask yourself the following questions:

- What are the sources/streams of my income at this time?
- What percentage of my practice and income comes from which market?
- Is my business base adequate to meet my income needs?
- What groups are lacking in my referral system?

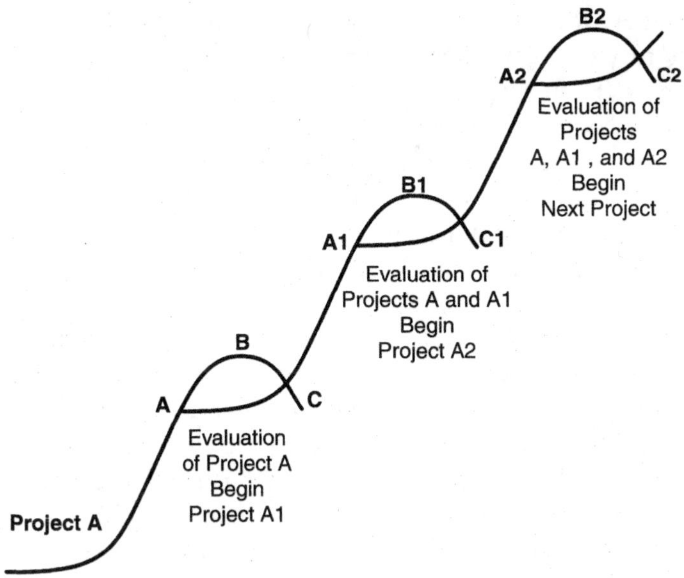

FIGURE 1.3 Example of a Sigmoid Curve

- What do I need to do to increase my income?
- What do I need to do to expand my income base?

Figure 1.3 is a developmental process model that supports your strategic marketing plan and encourages the skillful use of resources as you plan the next stage of your business future. "A" is the symbolic observation point at the beginning of the process and indicates where a different plan is to be put into effect. This is where you step back and evaluate "what is happening now." For example, perhaps you have met the goal for Year 1 or have not received as many referrals in the past few months as in prior months. This may be the point where you choose to send out a mailing to your referral sources. It could be about a new product or service, a training program you have taken, or so on. It is important to maintain visibility with your networking groups and to continue nurturing relationships you have made even as you move to the next stage of development.

At Point A, you also initiate a new developmental stage within the process. You may decide to begin a networking plan with another group of professionals. Then you begin anew with your strategic plan, developing materials for outreach to the new group.

"B" marks where a transition downward has begun. "C" indicates that the end is near. Point C is too late. Your goal is to keep your momentum moving forward by being attentive to the feedback from your plan. This process model is organic and dynamic.

Organize a marketing support group with other mental health practitioners and/or a mixed professional group. Connect, network, and build relationships as you grow your practice and increase your visibility in the community.

Participatory Partnership. Today's marketplace rewards collegiality, cooper-tition (combination of cooperation and competition), teamwork, diversity, sharing of information, strategic alliances, and time-limited, task-oriented partnerships. Participatory partnerships develop these qualities as well as the systemic reality of all business enterprises. Form teams with your colleagues or across professional disciplines, and offer programs and services to the wider community as well as the professional communities. Organize a marketing support group with other mental health practitioners and/or a mixed professional group. Connect, network, and build relationships as you grow your practice and increase your visibility in the community.

Developmental Practice. Building a practice is a developmental process. Your confidence and competency as a therapist play a role in your presentation of self, the products and services you offer, your referral systems, and the growth of your income base. Continually allow for a learning curve, start where you are, develop integrity with yourself in relation to your professional development phase, and plan for practice development and growth focused on the interplay between the present and your projected future.

Empiricism. Seek feedback continuously about your practice from the inner and outer systems. Inner systems relate to developing office methods for tracking income and expenses, sources of referrals, community trends, professional trends, and so on. The system is alive, dynamic, and interactive. This is the information age; knowledge offers the potential for deriving practice income. Outer systems include being in touch via professional newsletters and publications, local newspapers, issues of current clients, and so on. Whereas 5 to 6 years ago there were numerous behavioral managed-care organizations, more recently there have been several mergers and now 12 companies enroll 66 percent or 118 million of the 149 million enrolled in specialty behavioral managed-care organizations. If you are not on any of the panels listed and wish to have national managed-care companies as a component of your referral system, these would be the companies to target. The top 12, as of January 1997 are (*Open Minds*, May 1997):

Organization	*Enrollment in Thousands*
Value Behavioral Health, Inc.*	24,378
Merit Behavioral Care Corporation	18,585
Human Affairs International	15,898
Green Springs Health Services, Inc.	15,054
United Behavioral Health Care	11,307
Managed Health Networks	7,082
First Mental Health	6,000
MCC Behavioral Care, Inc.	5,733
Options Health Care, Inc.*	3,877
Family Enterprises, Inc.	3,498
CMG Health	3,309
Principal Behavioral Health Care	2,939

Referrals: Referrals are the lifeblood of your practice and your bank account. They require continual development. The following principles reflect the necessity of actively maintaining and tending to referral systems (Polonsky, 1992, p. 8):

- Referral sources are in constant flux; people leave, interpersonal conflicts develop, there may be downsizing, and so on.
- Maintain name recognition. Referral sources need to be kept informed and to have consistent reminders of your services and products. Develop a continuous marketing plan that includes mailing about new services/products, newsletters pertinent to their area of

Referral sources need to be kept informed and to have consistent reminders of your services and products.

*Options and Value Behavioral Health, Inc., merged the summer of 1998 to become ValueOptions and are now the second largest healthcare company in the United States.

interest, thank-you notes and/or telephone acknowledgments for referrals.

- A developed referral network will allow you to maintain professional and financial viability.
- If an economic downturn occurs, having a consistent marketing plan will give you a better chance of surviving and thriving.
- Marketing to referral systems is empowering and increases your sense of professional confidence and competency. Your mental health will be enhanced.
- The marketplace is a competitive one and having the appropriate credentials is not enough for survival. The appropriate credentials along with a business sensibility will greatly enhance your ability to remain in business as a mental health professional.

Behavioral healthcare is local and personal. At the same time, each individual is an organic part of ever-larger systems. At the global level, the larger system includes everyone and every institution. This is the holistic perspective from which we consider the mental health businessperson. We believe that we are interdependent and connectively related; movement is multidimensional throughout system levels and, to some degree, affects all within the system. This premise underlies our encouragement of mental health practitioners to perceive themselves as civic-oriented business professionals sharing the community with others. They need to strategically network with organizations and professionals at the local, national, and global level. Out of this perspective grows a flourishing, exciting practice.

An American Association of Marriage and Family Therapists survey found that 31 percent of those surveyed don't own or use computers in their practice. The computer is rapidly becoming necessary for the mental health practitioner. The computer via the Internet allows communication with colleagues around the world, and provides resources for the latest research about mental health. Many clients are informed consumers, who make use of Internet healthcare resources.

As a healthcare participant in the information age, think of communication in local, national, and global terms. Your clients will bring questions and/or material to you they have downloaded from a web site or online support group. People can now gather information in ways that level the playing field between the professional/expert and the client. If you haven't already done so, explore developing a web site for your products and services.

Communication has become multidimensional to a degree never imagined by professionals of past generations. Throughout the book, online sites are mentioned that are pertinent to your networking and referral opportunities. Technological adequacy for the mental health practitioner now includes a computer with Internet access as well as the ubiquitous answering machines, telephone/paging systems, the traditional written marketing materials, newsletters, and so on.

Communication has become multidimensional to a degree never imagined by professionals of past generations.

Summary

While you are highly educated and skilled, you may feel like an amateur when it comes to affirming and integrating the business side of being a mental health private practitioner. The word "amateur" means, "to love" and reflects doing what one loves without possessing a learned background in the particular area. While you may never learn "to love" the marketing side of business, you may begin to like it once you start practicing the techniques in the following chapters and develop greater confidence in your business skills.

Resources

Software

Genogram Software
The Computerized Genogram Company
780 Baconsfield Drive
Building 3, Suite 34
Macon, GA 31211
Telephone: (800) 634-8508 or (912) 743-2548
www.behavenet.com/humanware

Inspiration Software
Ceres Software, Inc.
P.O. Box 1629
Portland, Oregon 97207
(503) 245-9011

Internet

The Art of Business Web Site Promotion—Free downloads, a free newsletter, and an area for learning about site promotion and search engines can be found at this site. www.deadlock.com/promote

How to Announce Your Web Site—This text-only compilation and discussion of ways to promote web sites includes links to books on the subject. www.ep.com/faq/webannounce.html

How to Publicize a Web Site over the Internet—At this site, you'll find links to marketing sites plus a host of ideas for publicizing web sites at newsgroups, listservs, and search engines. www.samizdat .com/public.html

The Internet Marketing Center—Marketing, promotion, and advertising tips, strategies, and secrets can be found at this site. www.marketingtips.com

Kinko's—Free communication ideas from Kinko's. www.kinkos.com

Marketing Manager's Plain English Glossary—Here you'll find an explanation of web marketing phrases. www.jaderiver.com/glossary.htm

Marketing Topics—This collection of papers discusses the Internet and its impact on marketing. www.duke.edu/~mccann/mkttopic.htm

Mental Health Newsletter—Excellent resource and lists current hot mental health web sites. To sign up to receive free newsletter, send an e-mail to: mhn@cmhcsys.com

Northern Web Search Engine Tutorial—Designers can learn to build web pages that get noticed by the search engines. www.northernwebs.com/set

Office Depot—To download many resources for the small office. First click on "*Office Solutions*"; then click on "*Home Office Toolkit.*" Also, click on and check out their "*Small Business Handbook.*" www.officedepot.com

Promotion World—This site features an intriguing compendium of marketing tips, emphasizing free or cheap strategies. It also has "expert interviews" with marketing pros covering specific topics. www.promotionworld.com

The Postmaster—This is one of many sites that will, for a fee, submit your site's data to search engines, directories, and other sites that offer What's New and What's Cool areas. www.netcreations.com /postmaster

Ultimate Exposure—This site has a free web search engine/directory promotion page with links to other popular web locations where you can submit your site. www.turnpike.net

Organizations/Groups That Assist Small Businesses

The Atlantic Group Business Intermediaries
475 Hillside Avenue
Needham, MA 02494
Jim Kendall, Managing Director
(781) 444-0400
e-mail: dk756@aol.com
Offers small business consulting, business brokerage, and helps people start up businesses.

Flying Leap Productions
P.O. Box 23100
New Orleans, LA 70183
(504) 737-0089
(800) 449-3909 (call this number to receive a small magazine with materials about starting and growing a business.)
www.sb2000.com

Produces the PBS program "Small Business 2000." Their web site offers much free information and resources pertinent to small business owners.

National Association for the Self-Employed
c/o 2121 Precinct Line Road
Hurst, Texas 76054
Member Services: (800) 232-6273
www.nase.org

Small Business Administration (look up in the government pages of your local telephone directory).
10 Causeway Street
Boston, MA 02222-1093
(617) 565-5590
www.sba.gov

Networking Groups contact to see if there are networking groups in your area and/or how to begin one.

Business Network International
199 South Monte Vista, Suite 6
San Dimas, CA 91773-3080
(800) 825-8286
(909) 305-1818
www.bni.com

Le Tip International
4901 Morena Boulevard, Suite 703
San Diego, CA 92117
(800) 25 LE TIP
www.letip.com

ProfNet Inc.
702 East 25th Street
Erie, PA 16503
(800) 214-1999

Newsletters/Magazines

Business Spirit Journal
The Message Company
4 Camino Azul
Santa Fe, NM 87505
(505) 474-7604
Fax: (505) 471-2584
e-mail: message@nets.com
www.bizspirit.com

Computer Currents
Computer Currents Publishing
1250 Ninth Street
Berkeley, CA 94710
(800) 365-7773
Fax: (510) 527-4106
e-mail: editorial@compcurr.com
www.currents.net

The Inner Edge
101 Columbia
Aliso Viejo, CA 92656
(800) 899-1712
www.inneredge.com

InService: Continuing Education Opportunities for Counseling and Therapy Professionals
Publishing Services LLC
16659 East Hialeah Avenue
Aurora, CO 80015
(888) 690-5214
Fax: (303) 690-0093

Kettering Review
Charles F. Kettering Foundation
200 Commons Road
Dayton, OH 45459-2799
(513) 434-7300

Leadership in Action
Center for Creative Leadership
One Leadership Place
P.O. Box 26300
Greensboro, NC 27438-6300
(336) 286-4404
Fax: (336) 286-4434
e-mail: wilcoxm@leaders.ccl.org
www.josseybass.com

New England BOOMING
P.O. Box 1200
Boston, MA 02130-0010
(617) 522-1515
e-mail: info@nebooming.com

Open Minds: The Behavioral Health Industry Analyst
10 York Street
Suite 200
Gettysburg, PA 17325-2301
(717) 334-1329
Fax: (717) 334-0538
e-mail: openminds@openminds.com
www.openminds.com

Practice Innovations: Your Healthcare Network & Management Services Newsletter
c/o The Practice Sentry, LLC
83 Cambridge Street
Suite 2-D
Burlington, MA 01803
(781) 221-3180
Fax: (781) 221-3183

Practice Strategies, A Business Guide for Behavioral Healthcare Providers.
American Association for Marriage and Family Therapy
1133 Fifteenth Street, NW
Suite 300
Washington, DC 20005-2710
(202) 452-0109
Fax: (202) 223-2329

Self-Employed America
National Association for the Self-Employed
c/o 2121 Precinct Line Road
Hurst, TX 76054
www.nase.org
Member services: 800-232-6273

What's Working in Psychotherapy Practice Building
Practice Builder Association
18351 Jamboree Road
Irvine, CA 92612-1011
(714) 253-7900

Recommended Reading

Belenky, M.F., Clinch, B.M., Goldberger, N.R., & Tarule, M.M. (1986). *Women's ways of knowing—The development of self, voice, and mind* (Vol. 1). New York: Basic Books.

Bender, T. (1994, Winter). "The cultures of intellectual life." *Kettering Review* 46–52. Dayton, OH: Charles F. Kettering Foundation.

Berry, J. (Ed.). (1998, June/July). Fusion leadership: Unlocking the subtle forces that change people and organizations. *Business Spirit Journal: The Journal of Spirit at Work in Business, 7*, 7.

Blanchard, K., & Waghorn, T. (1997). *Mission possible: Becoming a world-class organization while there's still time.* New York: McGraw-Hill.

Bolles, R. (1996, March 1). Richard Bolles's secrets of finding a new job . . . a great new job. *Bottom Line Personal*, 9–10.

Boortstin, D.J. (1994, Winter). Democracy's secret virtue. *Kettering Review*, 16–20.

Boyte, H.C. (1994, Winter). Reinventing citizenship. *Kettering Review*, 78–87.

Bygrave, W.D. (1997). *The portable MBA in entrepreneurship* (2nd ed.). New York: Wiley.

Campbell, D.P. (1998). Down-to-earth life and leadership. *Leadership in Action, 18*(1) 14–15.

Cury, J.O. (1998, July). How to market your web site. *Boston Computer Currents*, 18–38.

Drucker, P.F. (1979). *Adventures of a bystander.* New York: Harper & Row.

Ferguson, T. (1997, November–December). Health care in cyberspace: Patients lead a revolution. *The Futurist*, 29–33.

Heim, P. (1993). *Hardball for women: Winning at the game of business.* New York: Penguin Books.

Hirsh, S.K., & Kummerow, J.M. (1987). *Introduction to type in organizational settings.* Palo Alto, CA: Consulting Psychologists Press.

Hopkins, M. (1998, August/September). In a "Healthy City," no one is superfluous. *The Inner Edge*, 1.

Jones, M. (1968). *Beyond the therapeutic community, social learning and social psychiatry.* New Haven, CT: Yale University Press.

Kamoroff, B.B. (1997). *Small-time operator: How to start your own small business, keep your books, pay your taxes and stay out of trouble!* (22nd ed.). South Bend, IN: And Books.

Keirsey, D., & Bates, M. (1984). *Please understand me: Character and temperament types.* Del Mar, CA: Gnosology Books.

Klein, H.L. (Ed.). (1997, August). Assessing the value of practice Websites: What works and what doesn't. *Managed Care Strategies, 5*(8), 6.

Landsbaum, M. (1998, July/August). Power networking: Boost your word-of-mouth advertising through referral organizations. *Self-Employed America*, 6–7.

Lawless, L.L. (1997). *Therapy, Inc.* New York: Wiley.

Lipman-Blumen, J. (1996). *The connective edge: Leading in an interdependent world.* San Francisco: Jossey-Bass.

McGoldrick, M., & Gerson, R. (1985). *Genograms in family assessment.* New York: Norton.

Morrison, R.M., & Stamps, R.F. (1988). *DSM-IV Internet companion: A complete guide to over 1500 web sites offering information on mental illness, keyed to DSM-IV.* New York: Norton.

Myers, I.B., & McCaulley, M.H. (1985). *Manual: A guide to the development and use of the Myers-Briggs Type Indicator* (Appendix D). Palo Alto, CA: Consulting Psychologist Press.

Oss, M.E. (Ed.). (1997, May). Questions healthcare marketers need to answer: Listening to the voice of the market. *Open Minds: The Behavioral Health Industry Analyst, 11*(5), 10.

Pascarella, P. (1998, June/July). Building corporate castles in the air. *The Inner Edge,* 5–8.

Pascarella, P., & Nagle, B.A. (1998). *Leveraging people and profit: The hard work of soft management.* Woburn, MA: Butterworth-Heinemann.

Palus, C.J., & Horth, D.M. (1998). Leading creatively. *Leadership in Action, 18*(2), 1–7.

Perry, P.M. (1998, January/February). Can newsletters make a sale? Yes, with these six techniques that motivate customers to read and buy. *Self Employed America,* 8–9.

Pilisuk, M., & Parks, S.H. (1986). *The healing web: Social networks and human survival.* Hanover, NH: University Press of New England.

Polonsky, I. (Ed.). (1992). *Managed care organizations, EAPs and PPOs Massachusetts 1992.* Oakland, CA: Professional Health Plan.

Polonsky, I. (1997, May). 19 percent increase in managed behavioral health enrollment. *Open Minds: The Behavioral Health Industry Analyst,* 12.

Radant, C. (1998, August). The new look for small business owners. *New England BOOMING,* 23.

Ronan, G.B. (1998, Spring). Profiles in productivity: Are you managing your practice or is it managing you? How successful therapists get down to business. *InService: Continuing Education Opportunities for Counseling and Therapy Professionals,* 4–5, 11.

Schaef, A.W., & Fassel, D. (1988). *The addictive organization.* San Francisco: Harper & Row.

Schön, D.A. (1994, Winter). The crisis of confidence in professional knowledge. *Kettering Review,* 21–28.

Scott, C.D., Jaffe, D., & Tobe, G. (1993). *Organizational vision, values and mission.* Menlo Park, CA: Crisp.

Senge, P.M. (1990). *The fifth discipline: The art and practice of the learning organization.* New York: Double Currency.

Sexton, D.L., & Smilor, R.W. (Eds.). (1997). *Entrepreneurship 2000.* Chicago: Upstart.

Sinetar, M. (1996). *To build the life you want, create the work you love: The spiritual dimension of entrepreneuring.* New York: Saint Martin's Press.

Steenbarger, B.N. (1997). *What the workforce numbers mean to you.* Syracuse, NY: SUNY Health Science Center.

Treadgold, R. (1997, September/October). Zen and the art of self-promotion. *The California Therapist,* 65–66.

Tuttle, G.M. (Ed.). (1997, December). Practice strategies: A business guide for behavioral healthcare providers. *Practice Strategies,* 3(12), 1–12.

Wallace, D. (1997, Fall). Tapping the potential of partnerships. *Update,* 8–9.

Wycoff, J. (1991). *Mindmapping: Your personal guide to exploring creativity and problem-solving.* New York: Berkley Books.

Wylie, M.S. (1998, January/February). Breaking free. *Family Therapy Networker,* 25–33.

Zobel, J. (1998). *Minding her own business: The self-employed woman's guide to taxes and recordkeeping.* Oakland, CA: Easthill Press.

Zuckerman, E. (1991). *The paper office: Forms guidelines and resources* (2nd ed.). New York: Guilford Press.

2

Strategic Niche Marketing

Chapter 1 helped you figure out what you wanted from your professional practice. This chapter helps you begin building your practice and assists you in meeting your professional goals. The key to having a successful practice is *marketing*. But the big questions are how and to whom? Successfully marketing your practice involves nine critical elements:

1. Identifying and assessing your market niche.
2. Finding the niche market needs.
3. Positioning yourself in the marketplace.
4. Presenting your products and services.
5. Creating a marketing strategy.
6. Designing a niche-specific marketing plan.
7. Creating a marketing budget.
8. Choosing communication vehicles.
9. Creating an action plan.

Once you complete these nine requirements, you can begin successfully marketing your practice.

Identifying and Assessing Your Market Niche

One definition of a "niche market" is a group of people or organizations with similar interests and needs.

Taking the Professional Practice to Niche Markets

During your training, you probably developed clinical specialties. A specialty serves as the launching point for a niche market, a small piece of a market segment. In fact, one definition of a niche market is a group of people or organizations with similar interests and needs. As a group, it can be clearly identified from other groups and subsequently to other groups. Ideally, your target niches should build on your professional interest and background. For example, a former school counselor trying to establish a professional practice might target parents of children with attention deficit hyperactivity disorder. The market segment is parents; the market niche is parents of children with ADHD. Therapists with a spiritual orientation might focus on building a practice in pastoral or transpersonal counseling. The more *strategic* you are in identifying your target group, the more successful your professional outreach will be. You are excluding some referrals, but you are focusing clearly on the clients who can best benefit from your special skills.

When you expand a current specialty or enter a new arena, you need to know the skills it requires. This understanding helps you design new services and products. When you identify a niche in which you have skills that meet the specialty's requirements, you have discovered gold. The following worksheet (Figure 2.1) helps you identify your market niche by looking at your professional mission and the expertise, specialties, and products you possess. Complete a Niche Market Characteristics Worksheet for each specialty and select the group/s you want to focus on. If you have identified more than one niche market, use the Niche Market Grid shown in Figure 2.2 to help you focus your efforts.

Assessing the Niche Market

To assess a niche market, you have to ask several questions, some of which require self-evaluation. Working with one niche at a time, ask yourself: "What is the history of this marketplace? What kinds of forces have created it?" When you know the history of the niche, you can use it to your advantage.

Next, think about the members of the market niche. What kinds of people will you come into contact with? What language do they speak? What are their values and beliefs? What general personality characteristics do the people in this niche have? You can evaluate a potential group by assessing the following conditions; then create a Client Profile of your market niche (see page 30).

To facilitate a good working relationship with the niche market, ask yourself: "Are the values and goals of this niche congruent with mine?"

Other aspects you need to consider are less tangible. To facilitate a good working relationship with the niche market, ask yourself: "Are the values and goals of this niche congruent with mine?" Since you will be

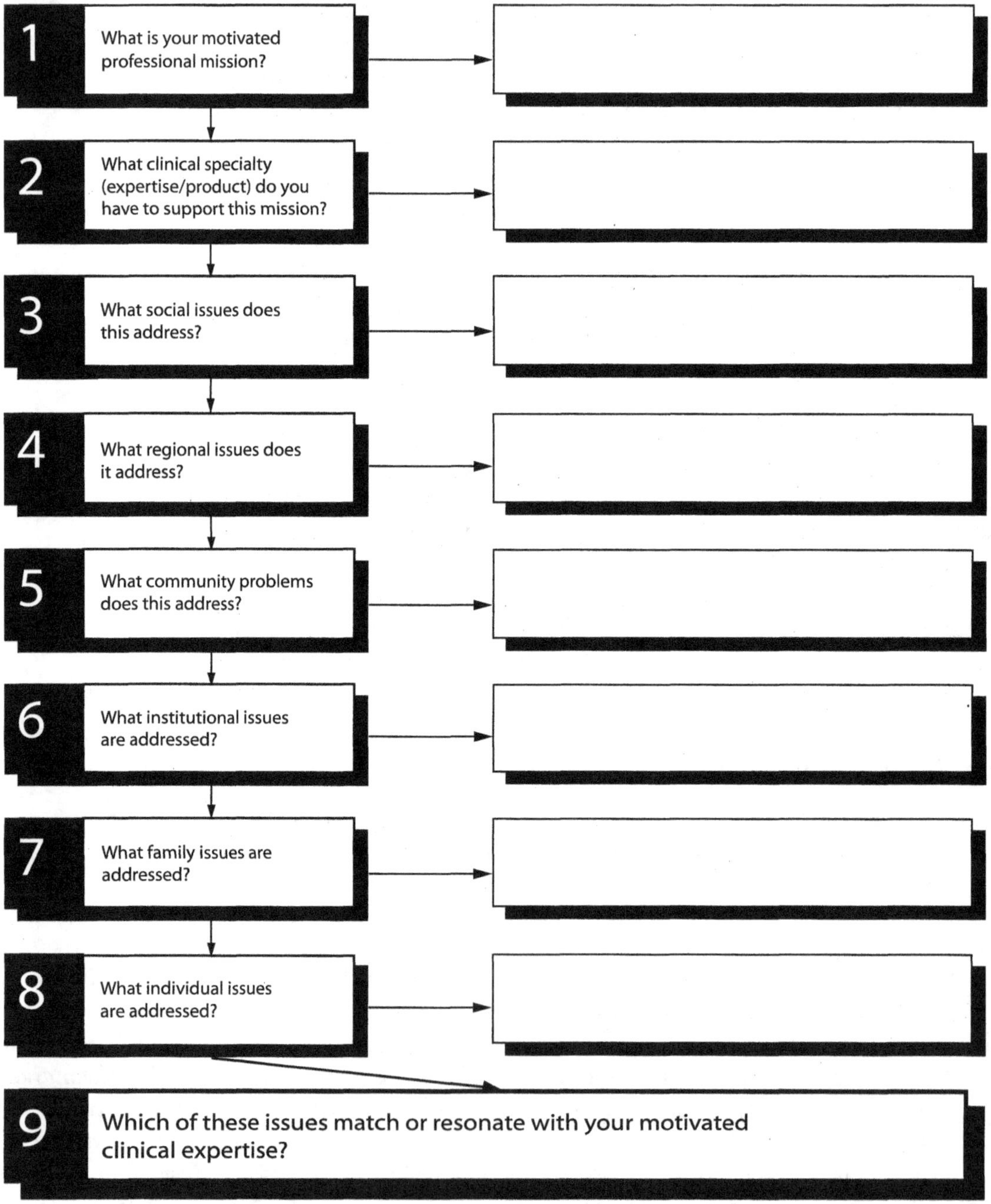

FIGURE 2.1 Niche Market Characteristics Worksheet

What phrase or term identifies members of this niche market?

1.

2.

3.

Rating Your Market Niches

Rate each one from 1-10 (1 = low/10 = high)	Niche 1	Niche 2	Niche 3
1. This niche market has money.			
2. This niche market will pay a premium for good service.			
3. There is a large population in this market.			
4. Competition in this area is low.			
5. I can easily get my information to the decision makers.			
6. I already have credibility with this niche market.			
7. The members of this market have a high **perceived** need.			
8. This market already knows they need what I offer.			
9. This niche market is in the right geographic area.			
Total Score			

Rate each niche market in every category from 1 through 10 and total them at the bottom. The niche market with the highest total score is the one with the highest potential for marketing success.

Using the Niche Market that scored highest, ask yourself the following questions:

What kind of information does this population value?

What personal experience do I have with this population and what has it taught me?

What important need(s) of this niche can I meet?

What services already exist to fill the need(s) of this marketplace?

Who would actually make the decision to purchase my services/products?

How can I best reach the decision maker?

Adapted from Lawless, L., *Therapy Inc.* (New York: John Wiley & Sons, 1997).

FIGURE 2.2 Niche Market Grid

Client Profile

Age group ____________________ Marital status ____________________

Average income ____________________ Size of household ____________________

Sex ____________________ Level of education ____________________

Geographic location ____

Reading or information gathering habits ____

____

____

Leisure activities ____

____

____

Special issues for this marketplace ____

____

____

Presenting problems/perceived needs ____

____

____

Inner or outer directed ____

____

working closely together, it is vital that you are working toward the same goals, using values that do not conflict. You also need to inquire about their experiences with other mental health professionals. It is helpful to know their encounters with, and their biases about your profession. Knowing their story allows you to expand their understanding. Similarly, what have your experiences with clients in this niche been like? When you examine your own biases, you are better equipped to avoid bringing them to your business dealings.

Current Trends

Another element to consider is current issues for this niche. For example, mental health professionals often struggle with managed care. What issues is your market niche currently dealing with? This information will help you match your skills to its perceived needs. What unidentified needs do you see in the market niche? After you have identified the issues, evaluate the potential of the market niche by asking yourself: "What are the current trends in the marketplace and the logical assumptions about how it will change?" Another way to analyze the future potential is to know the marketplace's history. You also need to be aware of the decision makers in the niche. For example, decision makers in mental health practice may include managed care companies, parents, counselors who refer clients, or employee assistance programs. Identify your niche market's decision makers and figure out how to reach them. You can waste many hours giving presentations to people who show interest, but cannot make a commitment. Spend your time wisely. It is not redeemable.

Spend your time wisely. It is not redeemable.

Finding your market niche also involves introspection. What kinds of services and products should you, and can you, offer? You need to examine your skills, developmental stages, and motivations. You wouldn't want to offer a service that you do not find interesting or challenging. Furthermore, with what kinds of individuals or groups do you work best? Identify the types of people with whom you are compatible. Ask yourself whether you want to work independently, with one other person, or with a group.

As you are preparing to enter a new marketplace, here are some more things to consider:

- What transferable skills do I have that are used and valued by this arena?

- What proof do I have of these skills (i.e., degrees, certification, and testimonials)?
- What experience have I had with this population?
- What specialized knowledge have I gained through my training and experience?
- How can I demonstrate my knowledge?
- Would I be considered an expert based on all the preceding areas?

You will be competing with others who have similar skills, experience, and knowledge. Be prepared to show how you are a better choice for the client's particular needs.

Finding the Niche Market Needs

By immersing yourself in the environment, you will quickly begin to recognize their needs and how they perceive them.

There are several ways to identify the needs of a niche market. Start by reading the newsletters and journals your niche produces, cruise their web sites, or attend one of their professional meetings or conferences. By immersing yourself in the environment, you will quickly begin to recognize their needs and how they perceive them. Then, ask yourself what kinds of services and products you can offer to fill their needs. If you have identified their needs, rest assured that others have also. Thus, you need to brainstorm how you can serve them in new ways. Look for voids in current services and develop innovative ways to fill them. You may see upcoming problems the market has not yet considered. It can help to create a list of short- and long-term goals for engaging your niche. This list can assist you in examining the needs of the group. The following are more ways to gather information about your niche market.

Assessing the Service Providers within the Market Niche

Begin with the Yellow Pages of your community and find the listings of services, benefits, and products for your niche market. If there are notable omissions, this may be the time to become creative in attracting your potential customers. Here are some other places to explore:

- *The Internet.* Look at different sites your potential clients might visit and find interesting. Check the links between each site. What is being offered? What is being said in the chat rooms or discussed in the news groups? These sites and discussion groups can offer a closer and more personal look than is ordinarily available.

- *Reading and Discussion Groups.* Do some brainstorming on your own and ask your local library if you can offer a book review group to discuss a topic that is important to your customers. See how it flies. Are the participants truly interested and able to talk about issues?
- *Community Forums.* Organize a community forum about your chosen topic. An excellent resource for setting up these groups is the Kettering Foundation National Issues Forums at (800)433-7834. You can also hold a brown bag lunch discussion group at your office. Offer a film that relates to a topic of interest and have a discussion afterward. A resource for mental illness videotapes is the Mental Illness Education Project Videos, telephone (201) 652-1989.
- *Contacts with Professionals.* Contact those who are offering services and offer to take them to lunch. Be thoroughly honest and curious. Many professionals will be generous with their time and eager to collaborate on outreach efforts.
- *Meetings with Businesses.* Talk to the administrators for the businesses and agencies that currently offer services to the population you are interested in. Find out what their biggest frustrations are with their work. Discover what services and products are being well received.
- *Libraries—Reading and Research.* Talk to your reference librarians. They can direct you to the publications that provide vital information about your marketplace. They can also request materials from other interlibrary sources that you may be unable to access in any other way.

Talk to your reference librarians. They can direct you to the publications that provide vital information about your marketplace.

Complete a market assessment of the service providers within the market niche. Answer the following five questions:

1. What services do they offer?
2. What products do they offer?
3. What do they charge?

4. Where are they located?
5. What services or products can be used in this market niche that are not currently offered?

Buying the products and attending any workshops or presentations offered by your competition will expand your expertise and provide more in-depth knowledge about what is already being marketed.

Presenting Your Products and Services

Many clients come in with a specific problem; after you listen to them, you can identify an underlying issue that supports current symptoms. When you talk to potential clients in the marketplace, the same kind of problem-solving process works: You need to be in dialogue with them about their underlying needs.

When you help potential clients identify foundational problems, they will be much more motivated to engage your services.

Defining the Benefits

When you help potential clients identify foundational problems, they will be much more motivated to engage your services. Frame what you do in terms of the benefit to them. Here are some typical "benefit statements" to weave into your conversations and outreach materials:

- Discover a safe place to talk.
- Improve your relationships.
- Find a referral source you feel good about.
- Better decision making.
- Increase your revenues.
- Successful team building.
- Reduce unnecessary costs.
- Increase your productivity.
- Reduced risk.

- Increase security.
- Prevent problems.

Clear communication of what you do and how it can help your target marketplace is the most critical part of professional outreach. This skill allows you to give clients what is most important to them—services and products that meet their needs.

Differentiating Products and Services

You must decide how to frame what you are offering, which means discriminating between products and services. Clients can understand products easier than they can recognize services. Products correlate to content and services to process. Products are clearly identifiable, while services are often difficult to visualize and quantify. An example of a mental health product is a stress management program, with a set curriculum, a workbook, and a fixed price. Stress management counseling is a service and has no fixed cost or identifiable material item.

Products are clearly identifiable, while services are often difficult to visualize and quantify.

When you design a product for a marketplace, you need to specify the need being served, and your applicable expertise and skills. The more precisely you identify any offering you propose to a marketplace, the easier it will be for your customers to commit to purchasing it. Now that you have zeroed in on the benefits of your services/products for the market niche, create descriptions of your business and its services/products. Expand your understanding of the benefits you plan to offer by writing the following business overview:

- *Executive Summary.* This includes information about your expertise, training, and experience as it relates to your niche market.
- *The Business.* Summarize the history of your business and how you have come to offer your services/products to this niche market.
- *Product/Service Summary.* Describe your product or service. This will help you crystallize your plan for offering these services and products.
- *Market Characteristics.* This summary should provide an overview of how your product/service meets the needs of today's marketplace.

Positioning Yourself in the Marketplace

Clients like stability and consistency of message.

Your name, logo, and trademark need to fit all the services and products you offer.

Positioning involves creating a context in the marketplace and placing your services in that context. Once you create a market position, it may be difficult to change in the public eye. There are many places to position yourself (i.e., prevention, clinical services, alternative services, and aftercare). Your position comes from your skills and how they relate to the overall market. Ideally, your niche will be in an underserved area that will continue to grow. Clients like stability and consistency of message. Maintain a string of continuity between the services and products you offer, never undermining your market position. Your name, logo, and trademark need to fit all the services and products you offer. Choose wisely in the beginning so that none of these have to change as your services and products evolve. For example, if you are targeting Parents of Children with ADHD, a service you could provide is "Dealing with Family Stress," since the ADHD diagnosis often creates a stressful family environment. Once you evaluate whether you want to be perceived as an MCO provider, traditional medical, or alternative medical provider, you can build your market approach. Figure 2.3 shows a sample positioning brainstorming process for reaching this decision.

Unique Selling Principle (USP) or You, Inc.

Every mental health professional works with some of the same business resources. There are a few hard assets and a few traits or soft assets that everybody shares or has in common. Most everyone has some sort of office setting to meet with clients; uses similar resources to network and research new contacts; shares the same goal to help clients; offers similar support systems or therapeutic approaches. However, many soft assets are particular to you and your personality, experience, and background. Once you sit down behind closed doors with a client, you are generally armed only with "you." So who are you professionally? What makes you unique? What do you bring to the table? Start right now to think of yourself as a "brand name"—*You, Inc.*—and how You differ from everybody else.

Write down the services and products that you offer. Read your list several times. Does it impress you? If not, do it again until it does. Start

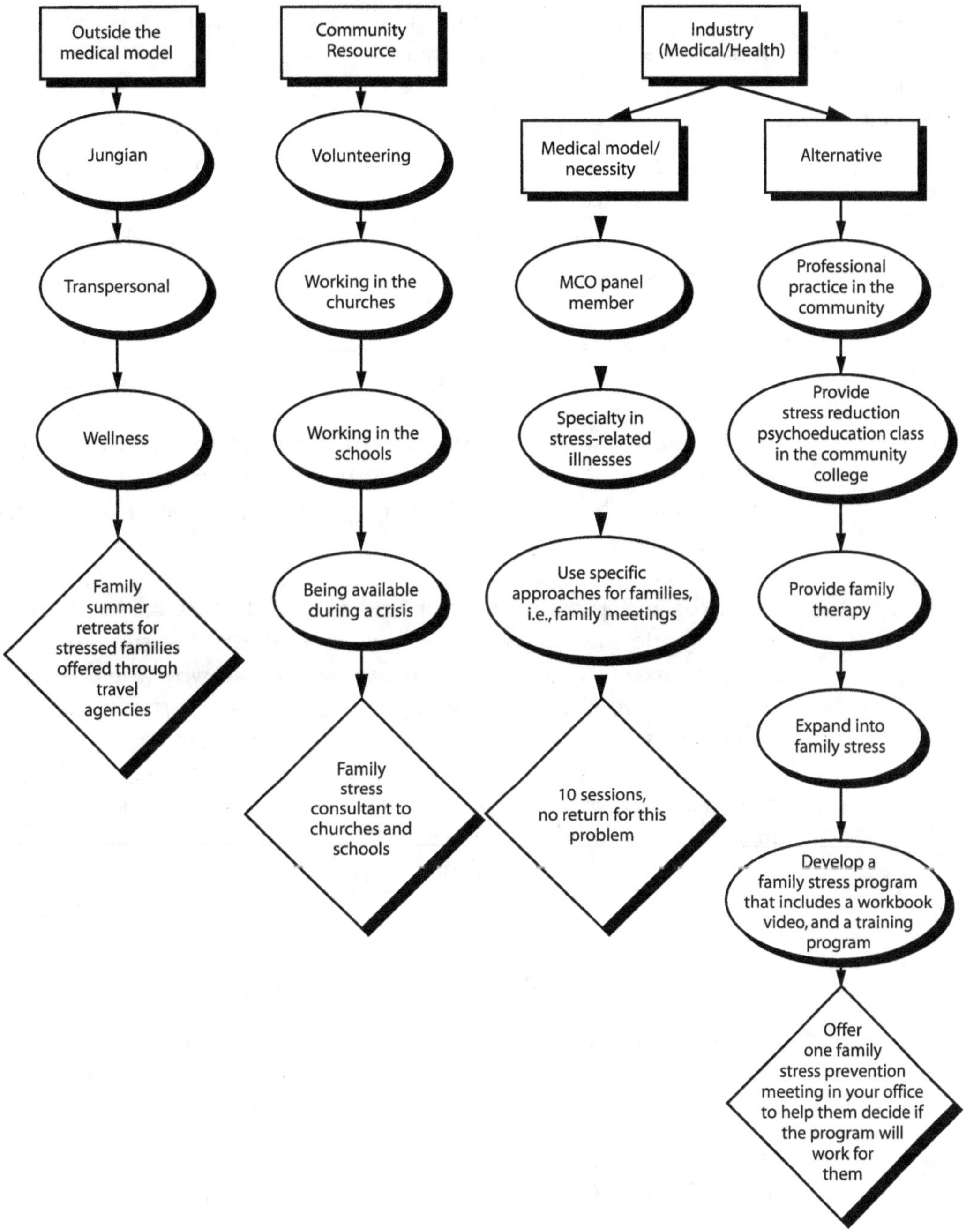

FIGURE 2.3 Positioning Family Stress in the Marketplace

Start by identifying all the qualities and knowledge that make you different from the therapists down the hall.

by identifying all the qualities and knowledge that make you different from the therapists down the hall.

- What have you done lately that they have not done?
- What would those therapists say is your greatest strength or your most impressive personal trait?
- How do these differences distinguish you from the rest of your profession?

As a professional, you probably have traits that other businesspersons may not have. Capitalize on those traits. Some of these traits could include returning phone calls quickly, listening to others effectively, delivering promised work on time, every time, being dependable, anticipating and solving problems before your customer is aware of them, saving clients money by averting crises, or completing projects within budget constraints.

To achieve success, you need to identify all your professional strengths and assets in your services and products. Compare your competitors' offerings to yours as well as their market position and costs. If someone had to choose between the two of you, why would the person choose you? Your market position and mix of services/products, needs to reflect the spirit of offering something unique, not of being competitive. For example, you can locate in another area and market to the people who are geographically closer. They would choose you because you are more convenient. No one is everything to everybody and there are always unique ways to distinguish you from others.

Creating a Marketing Strategy

You are probably already familiar with any specialty marketplace where you currently provide services. Before you commit more resources to expanding your clientele, do some market research.

Researching the Marketplace

Using your Client Profile and Market Niche worksheets, go to the library or search the Internet for information sources in this arena. Look at other service and product providers in the marketplace and see what they are offering clients and customers and how they are positioned. If you are comfortable with the concept, and it is ethical, focus groups can provide a wealth of information. An example would be a group consisting of parents of children with ADHD. A community focus group of these parents can tell you what services they are aware of, their perception of efficacy, and the needs they have that are not being served. The practice outcome evaluation is an in-house market research tool. What do your previous clients think about your services and products? The following resources may also be useful:

Look at other service and product providers in the marketplace and see what they are offering clients and customers and how they are positioned.

- Trade publications of other service and product providers.
- Competitor literature.
- Periodicals for consumers in the market niche.
- Government sources.
- Investor reports.
- Focus groups.

The *Practice Resource Directory* (Lawless, *Therapy Inc.*, John Wiley & Sons, 1997) is a valuable market research tool. As you gather information about the resources in your area for your clients, you are also finding out about the marketplace. When you inquire about community and professional resources, record the market research you believe is important on a Resource Directory Worksheet. Ask about the basics—name, address, telephone, contact people, services provided, costs of services and products, professionals involved, and clientele served. You might also ask about their future plans for their business, other resources they use, and what resources they still need to meet their clientele's needs. The following chapters include specialized Resource Directory Worksheets for each population addressed.

Engaging with the Marketplace

Once you have picked your niche and identified your unique strengths, you need to hone in on strategies to attract your potential clients. What can you offer the market niche? Think in terms of a range of services: workshops or trainings; wellness/prevention programs; groups—support or focus; psychotherapy—individual, couple, family, or child; consultation; or coaching. Do you have products such as audiotapes, videotapes, and train-the trainer programs? If not, could you create these products?

Designing a Niche-Specific Marketing Plan

Next, you must create a plan of action. Just as you might develop an individualized treatment plan for every client, you need to create specific marketing plans for your niche markets. Begin with a market overview and evaluate your market's stage of development. Every market niche goes through a life cycle: newly defined; growth; maturity; and end phase, if or when, the issue is resolved. There are opportunities and risk factors at every stage.

In the *newly defined stage,* the marketing approach includes psychoeducation. The risk here is entering an arena in which your potential clients may accept or reject your outreach. In the *growth stage,* potential clients have developed a clearer concept and context for their problem and communication is easier. The risk is greater competition. In a *mature market,* usually a few strong providers are dominant and can make it difficult to get a market foothold. These providers may lose touch with changing market needs or discontinue offerings that were not cost-effective. Such areas can open doors for the new, smaller provider. Finally during the *end stage* of a marketplace, demand is decreasing. This stage can provide opportunity for maintenance services and may point toward new products and services. This cycle is easily seen in the medical arena in relationship to polio. Once the vaccine was developed, the diagnosis reached its end phase, but many products and services were still needed by patients who were recovering from the effects of polio. In the mental health arena, the introduction of a new medication or treatment methodology can cause a market change.

Organize the activities in logical order and schedule outreach efforts for each stage, always allowing for constant refinement of your plan.

When you begin to develop marketing goals, we suggest starting at the outcome and working backward to what you can accomplish today. For example, if your goal is to receive more referrals from local physicians, brainstorm all the steps that would contribute to your success. Next, organize the activities in logical order and schedule outreach efforts for each stage, always allowing for constant refinement of your plan.

Figure 2.4 shows a Goal-Setting Worksheet for getting three referrals a week from parents of ADHD children.

After setting your goals and targeting completion dates, draw a map of the people who regularly come into contact with your niche market. Figure 2.5 illustrates a niche market universe map. Next prioritize the market universe in terms of the people you are most comfortable reaching out to, and then brainstorm about products and services you can create to introduce yourself. Be sure that you are very familiar with your market niche's lifestyle needs. This concept was developed by Stanford Research Institute (SRI) in California in the late 1970s and expanded further in *Therapy Inc*. (Lawless, 1997). Lifestyle marketing looks at the client as a member of a group: age, issue, values, needs, and tendency to be inner or outer directed. Your professional outreach needs to be designed to meet them where they feel most comfortable. The mindmap shown in Figure 2.6 illustrates the market universe and possible professional outreach for parents of children with ADHD.

The mindmap reveals several ways to reach your target market, such as public presentations, specialized workshops, and direct mail. These are the most common approaches. If you are comfortable with public speaking, the first two options present an ideal way to get your name out and reach your market. Potential audience members will see ads in local papers and notices in public places. Send invitations to niche market members and other professionals who provide ancillary services to this marketplace. For the direct mail marketing approach, a good "calling card" is a brochure tailored to the needs of your target market.

Pull all of this information together in a master marketing plan. The sample outline in Figure 2.7 will help you build your plan.

Choosing Communication Vehicles

In this chapter, we address the printed message. In later chapters, we deal with the spoken word and public relations. As outreach vehicles to develop your practice, they must be congruent. Every piece of paper you use in your business—stationery, brochures, business cards, and newsletters—contains a message, direct and indirect. As you create your market identity and position, everything you print needs to have a graphic

Today's date: 7/1/1999

!	My goal is: To receive 3 referrals per week for parents of children with ADHD	Completion date: 7/1/2000
1	What is the first step? Identify all the referral sources in my area	Target completion date: 9/1/1999
2	What is the second major step? Provide each with information about my specialty	Target completion date: 10/1/1999
3	What is the third major step? Schedule presentations about parental issues and solutions.	Target completion date: 11/1/1999
4	Next step: Design product/ workbook and audiotape for parents to use	Target completion date: 12/1/1999
5	Implementation: Professional outreach to niche market	Target completion date: 1/1/2000
6	Final step: Establish referral sources for overflow of referrals	Target completion date: 7/1/2000

FIGURE 2.4 Sample Goal-Setting Worksheet

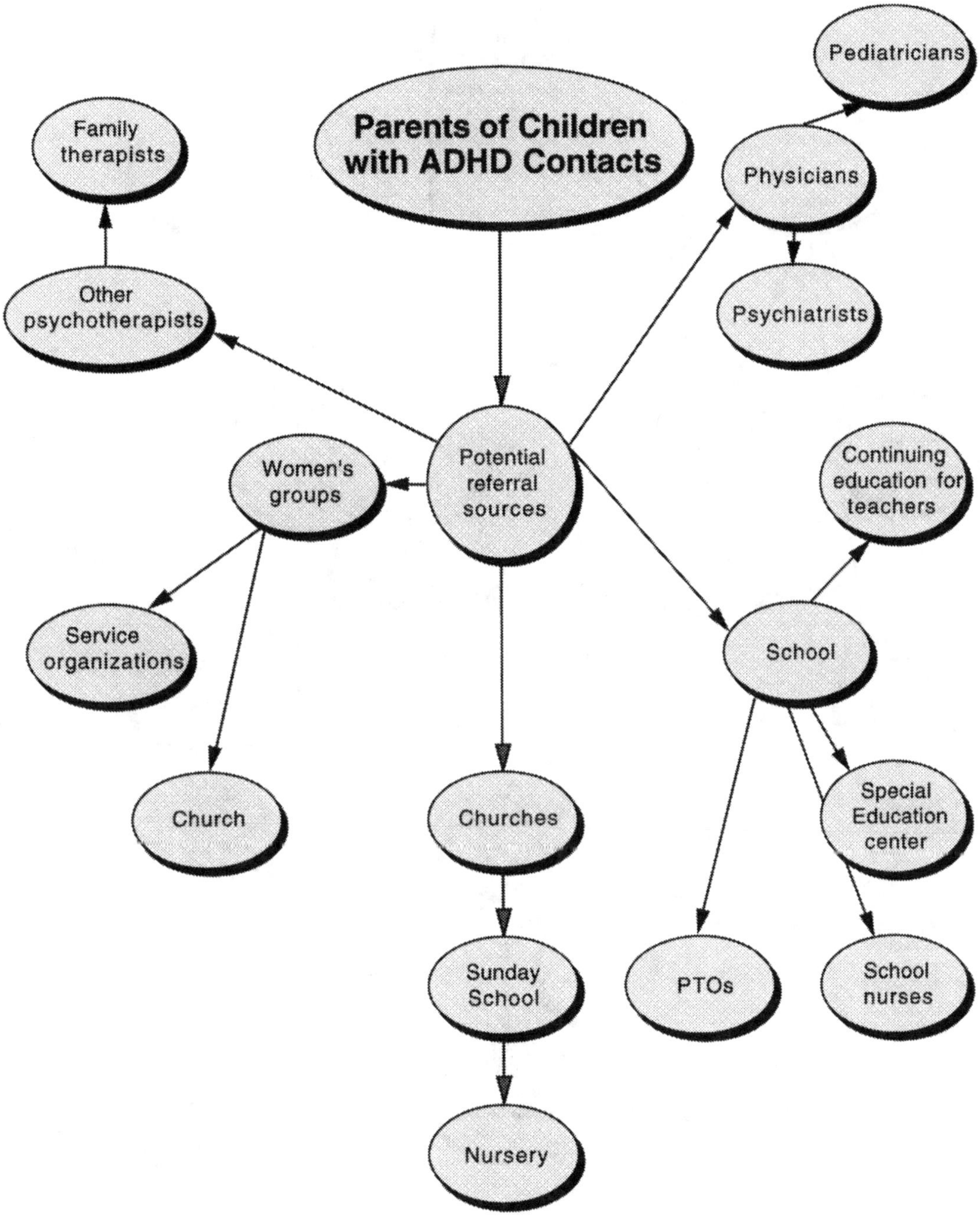

FIGURE 2.5 Niche Market Universe Map for Parents of Children with ADHD

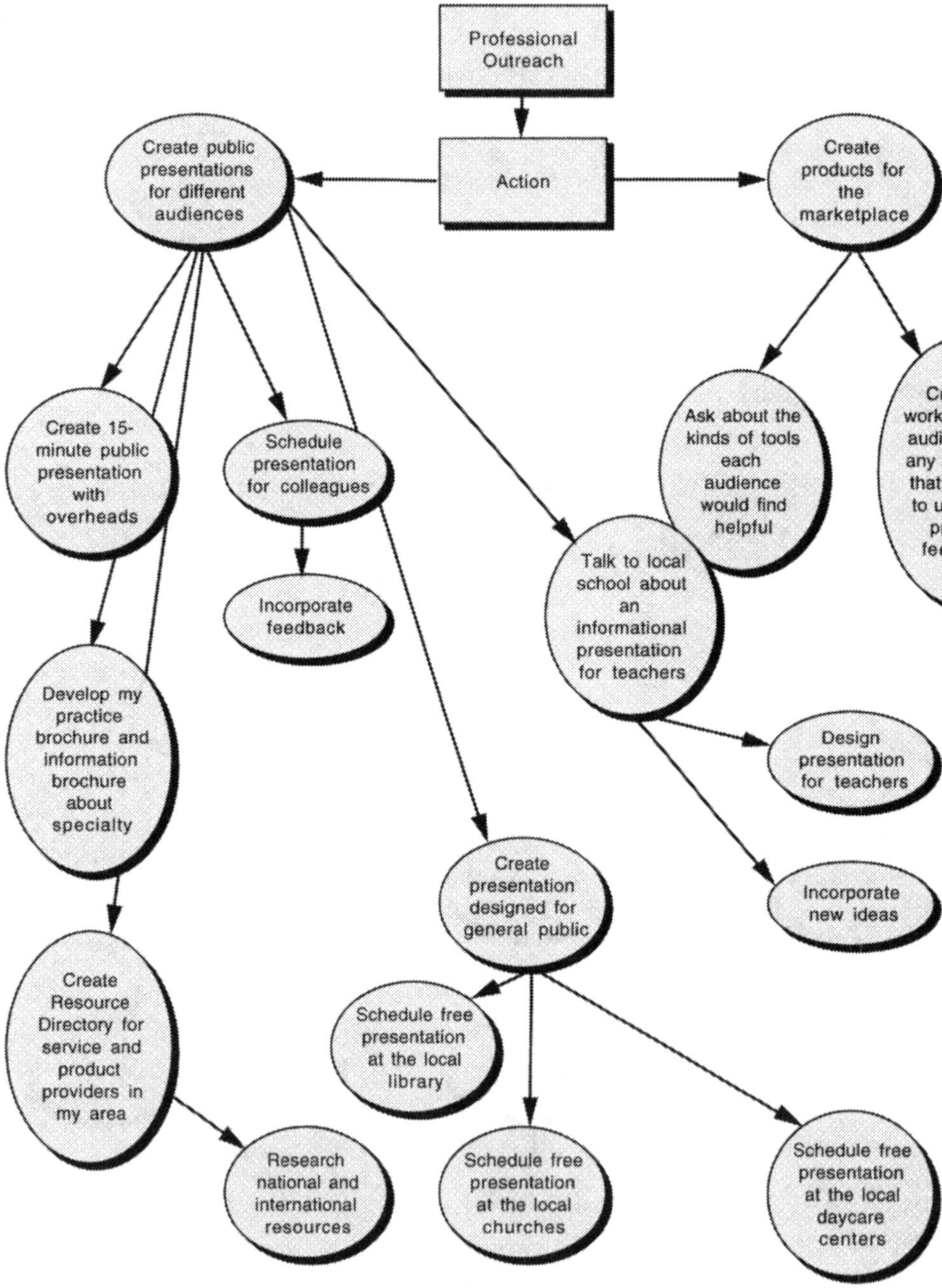

FIGURE 2.6 Professional Outreach Mindmap for Parents of Children with ADHD

What niche market are you identifying?

What is your marketing goal for this marketplace?

All the information that follows needs to be in relation to this niche market and the goal you have identified.

Executive Summary—You, Inc.

What is your professional developmental stage?

What is your personality type and how does it affect your work and the professional outreach approaches you can use successfully?

What is your story in relation to this market?

What is your motivation to enter this market?

What brought you to this marketplace?

What is your thread of continuity in this market?

How well are you prepared to enter this marketplace?

What is your motivated professional expertise?

What products have you developed?

What are your entrepreneurial skills?

Business Evaluation

What is your business structure's capability in terms of providing quality services to the niche market you have identified?

What resources are available (i.e., counseling, psychoeducation, consultation, products)?

Describe the psychoeducational workshops that can be provided.

How many groups can be held per month?

What is your travel availability per month?

How many clients can be seen per day/week?

Marketing Objectives

What is your personal definition of success?

What are your professional goals?

(Continued)

FIGURE 2.7 Marketing Planning Worksheet

Current Marketing Situation

What is the stage of development of this marketplace (new, growing, mature, ending/transitioning)?

What is the future of this market?

Niche Market

What are the characteristics of this market?

Who is the competition and what products and services do they offer?

What gaps in services and products exist?

What products and services can you provide?

Benefits
Your Unique Selling Position (USP)

Benefits
USP

Benefits
USP

For products and services that you duplicate with competitors, what benefit or USP do you have?

What products and services do you need to develop?

Outreach Strategy

What professional outreach do you currently have in place?

Advertising

Public relations

Professional relationships

Other

What is your current market position?

Traditional medical

Community resource

Alternative medical

Alternative general

Other

FIGURE 2.7 *(Continued)*

What is your specific position in your current market?

USP

Benefits

Pricing

Marketing Communications or Professional Outreach Plan

What outreach vehicles are best suited to your skills and the market's preferred interface?

What schedule suits your marketing approach?

What outreach efforts will you execute and when?

Date

Date

Date

Date

Date

Budgets

What will your plan cost?

$______

What percentage of your income can you commit to continuous marketing efforts?

______%

How will you ensure execution and maintenance of your marketing plan?

Keep a marketing journal that includes:

What you have done.

What you have avoided.

What was or was not successful.

Solutions to nonsuccess.

New ideas.

Join a marketing support group!

Should you hire a marketing consultant or specialized employee?

FIGURE 2.7 *(Continued)*

identity. When clients look at your newsletter, they need to see the same graphic style that you have on your brochure and business card. Your logo, type style, layout, and choice of words portray your graphic identity. You can create the basic examples in this book using desktop tools such as Microsoft Office™, or Claris Works™. Each of these desktop publishing packages has templates you can adapt to your needs. We have used templates from both. Preprinted color paper products from companies such as PaperDirect ((800) 272-7377) provide a 2–4-color layout for small print runs. When your budget allows, we recommend using a design service to enhance your outreach products. AdVentures at www.advenweb.com provides an example of high-quality outreach pieces.

Direct Mail

Break down your direct mail outreach list into four categories: "Known," "Knows of you," "Unknown with common interest," and "Unknown in target market."

Direct mail can be a successful tool if you use it wisely. Break down your direct mail outreach list into four categories: "Known," "Knows of you," "Unknown with common interest," and "Unknown in target market." The "Known" category includes people who personally know you and would open a mailer from you. The "Knows of you" group consists of people who have heard of you and might open a piece of mail out of curiosity. The "Unknown with common interest" are those who do not know about you but definitely have a common interest in the content of your mail, and the "Unknown in target market" group are those who do not know you and are only guessing that they might be interested.

Organize your mailing in this order: Known, Knows of, Common interest. Try never to venture into the last category unless you have a lot of money and can take the loss. Keep in mind the materials you mail will differ between categories. You can send the same brochure and return mail piece to everyone, but the cover letter should be different. The first cover letter, to the Known group, will be personal and seek their feedback or support. The second cover letter leverages off of the manner in which the recipients have heard of you. You are leading them to the reason you are reaching out to them. The third cover letter, Common interest, will speak to your common interest. Samples of these cover letters appear later in this book.

After you've organized the mailing, create your mailing lists in the following order:

- Personal lists of colleagues, friends, and acquaintances.
- Organizations you belong to.
- People who have attended your workshops or presentations.
- Yellow Pages listings in the areas of common interest.
- Publications you have published in.
- Publications that share your niche market interests.
- Public mailing lists such as professional licensees or specialties.
- Mailing list businesses where you can choose the demographics of your niche market.

Now that you have decided who will receive the mailers, what will you mail them? Your series of mailings could include an invitation to an open house at your office, along with a brochure and a business card. It could also include an announcement of a workshop or presentation, or an invitation to preview a new workshop. Some other pieces you can mail to your list include an invitation to subscribe to a newsletter, one free copy of the newsletter, or a free copy of the next issue of the newsletter with the option to no longer receive mailings if the person is not interested. Whatever you finally decide to send, be sure that each mailer contains a return postcard or Fax Back sheet to request more information, ask to be retained on the mailing list, or request removal from the mailing list.

A helpful tip for building your mailing list is to always get the mailing list or attendance sheet for any event you are involved in. Keep your lists in a database and record every time you send a mailer. Weed out the people who do not respond to your outreach ("seven strikes and you're out"). If after seven mailings, in a series of mailings, you have not received an interest response card, your final mailer should state that you will take the person's name off the list if you do not get a response.

Keep your lists in a database and record every time you send a mailer.

Advertising

Advertising is expensive and needs careful consideration. Each of the niche market chapters contains market-specific advertising information. Here are some basic layout rules to help make all your advertising pieces more effective.

Yellow Pages. If your business uses a business telephone line, this entitles you to list and advertise in your local and other regional Yellow Pages. The basic listing is free and any further advertising incurs a monthly fee. If you choose to use an in-line ad, make your copy easy to read and eye-catching. The parts of the ad include:

- *The Prehead.* Identifies what you are offering.
- *The Headline.* A larger print heading that identifies what you are offering in a larger scope.
- *The Subhead.* An elaboration of the head.
- *The Copy.* Continues to expand on your previous messages.
- *The Offer.* What you are offering to the public
- *Directions.* States how to contact you in a way that is safe and encouraging.

Figure 2.8 illustrates an effective Yellow Pages ad. There are many categories you can list under in your local Yellow Pages. You may have

A Community Mental Health Resource

The Alpha Centre

A Free Mental Health Resource Centre

If you have questions or concerns about your or your family's mental/emotional wellness, or if you want to understand this topic more fully, you are invited to use the Alpha Centre's free community resource center. The Centre includes books, audiotapes, and videotapes, informational newsletters and games that make mental health easy to understand. The Alpha Centre offers a safe place to find quality mental health services for individuals, families, and groups. Our goal is to create and support mental/emotional health, which in turn, we hope, produces a healthy, caring community.

Free Use of the Resource Center

No charge for a 10-minute informational consultation with a mental health professional that is completely confidential

Call The Alpha Centre .... @ 781.322.3051

6 Pleasant Street, #214, Malden MA 02148

FIGURE 2.8 Sample Ad in Yellow Pages

categories in your region that are not listed here. Some phone books also have an Internet guide. The following list was gathered from many regions:

Alcoholism Treatment
Career & Vocational Counseling
Clinics
Counseling Services
Counselors—Domestic Violence
Counselors—Family Relations
Counselors—Human Relations
Counselors—Personal
Crisis Services
Divorce Assistance
Drug Abuse & Addiction
Eating Disorders Information & Treatment Centers
Educational Consultants
Elder Care Consultants
Family Services
Gambling Abuse & Addiction Information & Treatment
Human Services Organizations
Marriage, Family & Child Counselors
Men's Organizations & Services
Mental Health Services
Mental Retardation & Developmentally Disabled Services
Motivational & Self-improvement Training & Materials
Parents' Guidance Instruction
Personology
Physicians (under the specialty of Psychiatry in the Physicians section)
Psychologists
Psychotherapy
Psychotherapy Information & Referral
Rehabilitation Services
Smokers' Information & Treatment Centers
Social Service Organizations
Social Workers
Speech & Language Pathologists
Spiritual Consultants
Suicide Prevention Counselors

Telecounselor
Telepsychologist
Women's Organizations & Services

Graphic Advertisements. The ad shown in Figure 2.8 would be much more interesting with an eye-catching graphic. If you do not have access to an affordable graphic designer, Dynamic Graphics ((800) 255-8800; www.dgusa.com) is a company you can subscribe to for copyright-free graphics.

There are also local tabletop publications where you can place a box ad or classified ad. These are generally weekly or monthly guides.

Posters. Posters are a common community announcement and are appropriate for the right market. You would not put a slick poster for a corporate workshop on an outdoor bulletin board, but you might tack up a notice for a Pet Grief support group.

Bulletin Boards. You need to match your offerings to the site you are posting at (e.g., book review at the library, lifestyle screening at the YMCA). Some sites you may want to consider for posting your notices are:

Sports equipment stores
Health fairs
Holistic centers
Health food stores
Employee bulletin boards
Community bulletin boards
Day care centers
Preschools
Middle schools
High schools
Community colleges
Universities
Vocational schools
Specialty schools
Supermarkets
Institutions
Libraries
Post offices
City halls
Senior centers
Hospitals

Your poster should have tear-off strips at the bottom to encourage interested readers to contact you. Figure 2.9 shows a poster with tear-off strips.

Metis

A Women's Therapy Group

come together to explore our unique strengths as women

Some concerns to be addressed:

- *Intimacy and relationships*
- *Recovering from divorce, loss, and trauma*
- *Communication skills and expression of needs*
- *Recognizing, breaking old habits that interfere with work, personal life*
- *Surviving in today's business world without sacrificing personal values*
- *Our feelings about our bodies and personal presence in the world*
- *Self-esteem – the daily challenge*

Groups forming now
eight-week commitment
$45 per session

Facilitated by:
Linda L. Lawless, M.A., LMFT
LMHC CGP

Call (781) 322-3051
for a personal interview

Metis 322-3051	Metis 322-3051	Metis 322-3051	Metis 322-3051	Metis 322-3051	Metis 322-3051	Metis 322-3051	Metis 322-3051	Metis 322-3051

FIGURE 2.9 Sample Poster with Tear-Off Strips

Informational Pieces

The bottom line in any informational piece is information that is accurate, timely, and tasteful.

Newsletters and Brochures. Informational pieces include brochures, newsletters, and public speaking presentations. In the following chapters, we have used the National Institute of Mental Health's (NIMH) copyright-free information. For more general informational content we recommend First Draft. They provide timely, interesting information that you can use for the general public. They can be reached at (800) 878-5331. The newsletter for MCO employees, in Chapter 7 was taken from this source. The best solution to copyright problems is your original work. If you do not want to create your own newsletter, you can order prepared copies with your information printed from Human Services Publications at (800) 873-2834. The bottom line in any informational piece is that your information is accurate, timely, and tasteful. Whenever you present an outreach piece, make certain you never imply that the audience in any way should take the information personally, as if they have a mental illness or specific problem.

Technology—The Internet

The Internet is a potential networking and referral source that attracts many people who are highly educated and want to be in control of their well-being.

Although the Internet still may seem big and mysterious, it is a rapidly expanding marketplace with many resources and opportunities for mental health professionals. It lies between the written and spoken word since people can access it as text only or can add video and sound. This information is meant to get you thinking about marketing on the Internet and asking yourself if it is a good media for you. We recommend using the Internet, first, as an informational resource. Many sites offer information that can benefit you and your clients. Second, the Internet is a potential networking and referral source that attracts many people who are highly educated and motivated and want to be in control of their well-being. You can reach this population via referrals from other people's web pages or via your own web page. Internet resources are listed at the end of this chapter in the Resource section. Rather than list hundreds of Internet sites, we have listed resource sites that can bring you to the sites that interest you. If you are concerned about the ethical aspects of Internet, a professional association for ethics online began in 1997 and acts as a central coordinator for mental health activity and advocacy. The International Society for Mental Health Online web site is www.ismho.org.

To easily use the Internet, you must have a computer with a modem and subscribe to an Internet Service Provider (ISP) such as America Online or CompuServe. Talk with friends about their equipment, consult a professional in the field, do some real-time trial runs, and then make your own decisions. You can initiate your Internet presence by listing on several sites that offer professional referrals, then graduate to your own web page. To begin to get referrals from Internet sites you will need an e-mail address, which is easily obtained through your ISP.

Your directory listings need to be stated in a way that your target audience can easily understand. Are you pitching to colleagues or potential clients? A simple paragraph can be very different for these populations. Your colleagues will accept "psychobabble" and *DSM-IV* terminology. Not so, the general public. Your Internet messages need to be comprehensible to the layperson and structured like your other "benefit-oriented" outreach.

Next, determine the objectives for your site. One objective could be to position yourself as an expert in a particular specialty. You can offer your services and products, link to related sites, offer an ordering service for related books and other media, and have a chat room where colleagues talk about their work and ask questions. A consumer site could offer similar resources (e.g., information, links to related sites, an ordering service, chat room) but the content would be considerably different. You cannot serve the needs of both with the same information. You can split your site into "professional services" and "consumer services," but know that most consumers will visit both. Decide what you want to get out of your Internet presence. Do you want visibility, validation, clients, or networking with other professionals? Your goal should be measurable so you can decide after 6 months of Internet expense whether it is paying off.

You can offer your services and products, link to related sites, offer an ordering service for related books and other media, and have a chat room where colleagues talk about their work and ask questions.

Set a budget. Your budget can range between $19.95 or less for an ISP subscription and e-mail address to thousands of dollars for a web server and subsequent advertising. Now is the time to do some comparison-shopping. Surf the net and look at web pages. Which ones do you like? Who produced them? What did they cost? What do the different aspects of the page cost? What are your advertising options? Some feel that "hotlinks" are effective advertising, while others want flashing banner ads (a picture strip that contains images and text and is located at the top of web pages). There is also key word advertising. This means listing key words with web search engines so that when users type in "mental health," your web page is listed.

Study your advertising options. Advertising on the Internet can be costly. If you are moving into banner ads and animated graphics, you are venturing into a more sophisticated advertising medium that requires expertise, time, and money. Use a competent Internet consultant to guide you through this maze.

There are many resources for entering this medium. The ones we have found most user friendly are the books whose titles start with *An Idiot's Guide To . . .* For the Macintosh platform, the books by Robin Williams are listed under Resources at the end of this chapter. Robin Williams also has a CD-ROM entitled Home Sweet Home Page and the Kitchen Sink that helps you set up your home page on the Internet. Like her books, it is very user friendly. All her publications are available through the PeachPit Press at (800) 283-9444 or (510) 524-2178; Fax: (510) 524-2221; www.peachpit.com.

The Internet explosion is much like the transitions that occurred with the invention of the telephone and the steam engine. Many spin-off industries have emerged. The future of the Internet and its potential to promote mental health are yet to be fully discovered. Avoid quick superficial self-assessments and misinformation, and explore the ramifications of having information about mental illness and mental wellness available to everyone. On the Internet, people with valuable resources are easily located, and professionals can dialogue about new ways of helping their clients.

Direct mail costs money. Donating your services for free public lectures costs time. Both time and money are spent wisely if they result in referrals.

The technology to create interactive programs is there for you to use. The CD-ROM and DVD technology provides the opportunity to create interactive workshops for professionals and psychoeducational programs for clients. Once the program has been created, the cost of reproducing each CD-ROM can be as low as one dollar. There is a learning curve for the design software, so you may want to find someone to do the work for you. A cross platform (works on both MS-DOS and Macintosh) software program is Director. When you are ready to mail out your CD-ROM, you will need "jewel" cases or you can order colorful envelopes from a company called Press Kits ((508) 660-2020).

Creating a Marketing Budget

Direct mail costs money. Donating your services for free public lectures costs time. Both time and money are spent wisely if they result in referrals.

If you are going to be in a business, as all therapists in private practice are, you need to establish a considerable yearly marketing budget.

You need to establish a considerable yearly marketing budget.

Money. You can spend as little as 5 percent and as much as 50 percent on your marketing costs. I suggest something in between, say 25 percent, *every month.* If your current operating budget is $0, then you will be largely working out of your start-up budget. When you are starting up, you will use a higher percentage of money for outreach, maybe 50 percent or more. However, after you have settled in and have started making referral contacts, your marketing budget should gradually decline until you reach your target percentage for each month.

Time. You can consume a lot of time marketing your practice and getting referrals, and your time is just as precious as your money. You can use your time for many kinds of professional outreach activities. Before you sign up to be treasurer or newsletter editor for a new group, ask yourself where you want to make strategic connections. Also, ask yourself what percentage of your time you should use for outreach. Invest your time in the areas that will serve you effectively.

Before you sign up to be treasurer or newsletter editor for a new group, ask yourself where you want to make strategic connections.

Choosing Your Tools. Your tools need to support what you can do. Don't set up a public speaking project if speaking in public terrifies you. Direct mail may be a better selection for you, even if it has a lower return on investment, because you will actually do it. After you have decided on the tools you know you will put into action, make a budget list, as shown in the following example:

Tool	*Cost per Use*	*Frequency*	*Monthly Cost*
Direct mail	$200	Monthly	$200
Newsletter ad	$150	Quarterly	$ 50
Total			$250

Tool	*Time Cost per Use*	*Frequency*	*Monthly Cost*
Public speaking	6 hours	Quarterly	2 hours
Byline	4 hours	Monthly	4 hours
Professional committee	6 hours	Quarterly	2 hours
Total			8 hours

Income. Fee setting is another difficult issue for many professionals. When you find yourself struggling to state your hourly rate, think of all the time, money, and personal work you have put into becoming what you are today. Aren't you worth an honest sum? Develop a system for fee negotiations. Know what you charge for the services and products you offer. You may work on a sliding scale but at least know the circumstances of your nonclinical clients. In this arena, you can negotiate and exchange things such as use of their mailing list or advertisements in their newsletter. It is very important to know when, what, and how you negotiate.

Have a letter of agreement or contract in writing. Figure 2.10 shows a sample letter of agreement to provide a workshop. In addition to creating a letter of agreement or contract, bill professionally. If your client has a preferred reimbursement form, use it. If their form does not include your fees or where they should be sent, include them. If you charge interest on balances due after a certain number of days, make that clear on your invoice and in your contract. Know and abide by your professional association's code of ethics.

When you move outside the framework of an individual paying an hourly fee, you need to look at new ways of equating your services and products. Don't assume anything. State in writing everything you will offer and everything the client expects. Sometimes a simple sample letter of agreement is all you need. Other times a detailed proposal and contract is necessary. Do all the things a good businessperson would do. Your contract should specify whatever you have agreed to do, and what you will not do.

Creating an Action Plan

Review your potential client reactions and revise anything that appears to be unclear or bland.

Your marketing dialogue or "dialectic marketing" refers to your responses to inquiries that result from your professional outreach. Review your potential client reactions and revise anything that appears to be unclear or bland. You must communicate who you are and what you do (Authentic Marketing) in a way that attracts and motivates your target market to develop a professional business relationship with you.

Continuous Marketing

On an organizational level, keep a tickler file for following up on leads and responses. This maintains a continual flow between you and your niche market, and keeps your contacts up to date. Always maintain

Alpha Centre

6 Pleasant Street Suite 214 Malden MA 02148 781-322-3051

Our mission is to be a professional resource in support of the health and well-being of
- The whole person
- Families
- Businesses, institutions, and
- Municipalities

in the service of creating caring community

Our services include psychoeducational workshops on:

EATING DISORDERS

HOW TO CHOOSE THE RIGHT THERAPIST

SELF-ESTEEM AND HEALTH

PARENTING TRAINING

COMMUNICATION SKILLS AND CONFLICT MANAGEMENT

STRESS MANAGEMENT

MEDIATION

BEING A SUCCESSFUL SINGLE

SURVIVING AND THRIVING AS A STEP-FAMILY

FAMILY MEETINGS

MENTAL ILLNESS - WHAT IS IT?

SUCCESSFUL AGING

SUCCESSFUL LIFESTYLE CHANGE

Linda L Lawless LMHC LMFT and the ______________________

It is agreed that Ms. Lawless will pr ovide a six hour training workshop on Saturday October 14. The two themes to be covered are: The World of Managed Care and Building a Practice in the Managed Car e World. She will arrive on the Friday evening prior to the workshop and leave on the Sunday morning after the workshop.

The contractor ____________________ agrees to: pay for the following:

- Ms. Lawless's travel expenses to and from Topeka, Kansas,
- Lodging such as a Holiday Inn or equivalent lodging for the evenings of October 13 and 14,
- Daily meal charges, with a maximum or $40,
- Transportation to and from the airport in Boston and Topeka, and to and from the hotel to the workshop location.

Half of these expenses will be paid to Ms. Lawless upon agreement to these provisions and the balance within two weeks of her providing the training.

Any changes in this agr eement must be made in writing and agreed to by both parties.

Signed: Linda L Lawless LMHC LMFT ______________________________

Date:

The Representative for the contractor ______________/

____

Position:______________________________________

Date:

FIGURE 2.10 Sample Letter of Agreement

communication, whether it be a brief note or a carefully planned newsletter. Any occasion can be an opportunity to reach out to the marketplace. You can send out thank-you notes, mail letters welcoming new businesses, invite them to events or open houses, announce community service projects, or congratulate a colleague's achievement—these are all gestures that strengthen your relationship with your niche market. They open a dialogue for learning and exchanging information.

Marketing support groups are another good way to find creative ideas, try out new outreach approaches, and get support for your activities.

Marketing support groups are another good way to find creative ideas, try out new outreach approaches, and get support for your activities. Some professional associations offer help in setting up groups. If a group is not available in your area, start your own or contact a practice consultant for a referral.

Keep a record of all your professional outreach efforts in your marketing activity journal. This will help you see how many things can be thought of as marketing, as well as their relative effectiveness. Include meetings where you discuss your work, your contacts with managed care employees, and the help you gave a colleague who called in a crisis. All these events communicate what you do and the value of your mental health skills, services and products. The following sample marketing journal format records the responses received from individual activities:

Date of Entry	*Event*	*Project*	*Contact*	*Follow-Up*	*Complete*
1-1-2000	Received FAX Back Sheet	Women's Group	Peter Jones	1-2-2000	1-2-2000
1-9-2000	Presented @ networking breakfast	Supervision Grp	See mailing list	1-16-2000	1-18-99
1-16-2000	Submitted ED article to magazine. Starting a byline	Individual Clients	Sue Smith	2-28-2000	
1-17-2000	Sent PCP Release for New Client	Individual Clients	Dr. Brown	1-24-2000	

Right and Wrong—The Ethical Considerations of Marketing

Mental health professionals obviously should not try to change people's behavior through unethical behavior. But just where do they need to draw the line on efforts to penetrate a marketplace? The basics are to tell the truth and give a fair value for your services and products. The following ethical guidelines are a synthesis of the ethical guidelines for licensed mental health professionals (Corey, Corey, & Callanan, 1998).

Some mental health professionals have taken the stance that advertising or marketing is unethical and is not permissible in any shape or form. Our view is that it is unacceptable to conduct any marketing effort that can be construed as dishonest, or an abuse of power. Professionals must always accurately represent their education, training, licenses, experience, and subsequent specialties in any outreach piece or event. If anyone else misrepresents any of this information, professionals should take action to correct it. They should never pay a media employee for inclusion in a news item. Any paid advertising or outreach piece needs to be identified as such unless the format and content make it obvious. Testimonials should not be solicited from current or former clients, who might be susceptible to undue influence. Direct mail pieces or phone calls should not be made to current or prior clients unless they have previously indicated it is all right to do so. This means that during the intake or exit interview the client should sign a statement that approves of this future contact. Public presentations or written articles that include information about any kind of mental illness or emotional problems must never infer that any member of the reading or listening audience should take it personally.

Professionals must always accurately represent their education, training, licenses, experience, and subsequent specialties in any outreach piece or event.

We approach professional outreach from a psychoeducational perspective: you are giving people information and experiences that they can use to make informed decisions about products or services that you offer. We even go a step further in citing the moral imperative of letting the community know about your skills so that the people who are in need will have access to services that can help them.

The American Marketing Association's Code of Ethics is congruent with ethical marketing. Their code states, " Marketers must accept responsibility for the consequences of their activities and make every effort to ensure that their decisions, recommendations, and actions function to identify, serve, and satisfy all relevant publics: customers, organizations and society" (Bartlett, 1998).

We hope you can comfortably make honest, ethical, authentic professional outreach a part of your future professional success.

Summary

In this chapter, we introduced the keys to successful marketing: identifying a clear niche, understanding your customers' needs, being able to communicate the benefits of your services and products to meet their needs, making sure the customer knows your market "position," creating a market strategy, establishing month-by-month plans and timetables, understanding your budget, and drawing up a realistic action plan.

Now you must implement market-specific detailed outreach and marketing plans for your chosen niche and get those referrals. The following chapters provide marketing strategies to help you decide which niches fit you best, and samples to aid you in developing your referral sources.

Resources

Community Forums

Kettering Foundation (800)433-7834

Mental Illness Education Project (201)652-1989

Desktop Publication

Ad Ventures—www.advenweb.com

Dynamic Graphics (800)255-8800/www.dgusa.com

Paper Direct (800)272-7377/Human Service Publications (800)873-2834

Internet

The International Society for Mental Health Online—www.ismho.org

The Mining Company—www.miningco.com/ and search on mental health.

The Clinician's Yellow Pages—www.cmhc.com/cyp/

The Mental Health Page—www.licensure.com/trlinks/links.html

The American Psychological Association—www.apa.org/homepage.html

The AMA Web Guide to Psychiatry Related Sites—www.ama-assn.org/public/journals/psyc/webguide.htm

The American Psychiatric Association—www.ama-assn.org/home.htm/

The National Institute of Mental Health (NIMH)—www.nimh.nih.gov/
American Association of Marriage Family Therapists (AAMFT)—www.aamft.org/
The National Board of Certified Counselors—www.nbcc.org/
National Association of Social Workers (NASW)—www.naswdc.org/
The American Mental Health Counselors Association (AMHCA)—www.amhca.org/index.html
At Health—www.athealth.com/prointro.html
Behavior Online—www.behavior.net/guides/index.html
PsychLink—www.psychlink.com/
The Department of Health and Human Services—www.hhs.gov/index.html
Psychology—www.princeton.edu/~harnad/psyc.html
Mental Health Home Page—www.mentalhealth.com
Mental Health Net—www.cmhc.com
Yahoo Government—www.yahoo.com/Government/ and search on mental health

Multimedia

CD-ROM—Williams, R., & Mark, D. (1997). Home Sweet Home Page and the Kitchen Sink (Vol. 1997): PeachPit Press.
Press Kits (508)660-2020

Software Development Packages

Director
Dreamweaver
GoLive CyberStudio
Adobe PageMill
Microsoft FrontPage

Newsletter Copy

First Draft—(800) 878-5331

Videotapes on Mental Health/Illness

Mental Illness Education Project Videos—www.miepvideos.org
At-Risk Resources—www.at-risk.com

Recommended Reading

Ackley, D.C. (1997). *Breaking free of managed care: A step-by-step guide to regaining control of your practice*. New York: Guilford Press.

Bartlett, F. (Ed.). (1998). *Marketing builder.* Washington DC: JIAN.

Browning, C.H. (1984). *How to build a practice clientele using key referral sources—A sourcebook*. Los Alamitos, CA: Duncliff's.

Corey, G., Corey, M.S., & Callanan, P. (1998). *Issues and ethics in the helping professions* (5th ed.). New York: Brooks/Cole.

Crandall, R. (Ed.). (1997). *Marketing for people not in marketing*. Corta Madera, CA: Select Press.

Davis, J. (Ed.). (1996). *Marketing for therapists.* New York: Jossey-Bass.

Grand, L. (1998). *The free agent therapist.* Barrington, IL: The Free Agent Therapist.

Heller, K.M. (1997). *Strategic marketing: How to achieve independence and prosperity in your mental health practice*. Sarasota, FL: Professional Resource Press.

Hiebing, R.G., & Cooper, S.W. (1997). *The successful marketing plan* (2nd ed.). Lincolnwood Chicago: NTC Books.

Lawless, L.L. (1997). *Therapy Inc.: A hands-on guide to developing, positioning, and marketing your mental health practice in the 90s.* New York: Wiley.

Miriam Ottee, M. (1998). *Marketing with speeches and seminars: Your key to more clients and referrals.* Seattle, WA: ZEST Press.

Putman, A. (1990). *Marketing your services: A step-by-step guide for small businesses and professionals.* New York: Wiley.

Smith, J. (1995). *The new publicity kit.* New York: Wiley.

Williams, R. (1994). *The non-designer's design book: Design and typographic principles for the visual novice*. Berkeley, CA: PeachPit Press.

Williams, R. (1996). *Beyond the MAC is not a typewriter.* Berkeley, CA: PeachPit Press.

3

Strategies for Getting Referrals from Physicians

Physicians are often the gatekeepers for mental health services and sometimes seem to be one of the "bad guys" in the managed-care transformation of the mental health field. Physicians, however, have suffered as much as, if not more than, mental health professionals, in terms of losing control of their profession and experiencing reduced income in the managed care marketplace turnover. Physicians can be "good guys"—collaborators and professionals—who also benefit from an integrated healthcare system that includes mental health.

Since physicians often have the power to refer and approve treatment, mental health professionals have traditionally focused on this referral base. These referrals can still be an excellent resource for psychotherapists, but such referrals have diminished as many physicians have joined group practices, which tend to refer to other practice groups. Physicians in group practices often can only refer to panels of mental health professionals identified by the patient's MCO, or to the hospital or group where the physician works or has a contract. Today's mental health professional needs to think of physicians as collaborators in the overall treatment of patients.

Physicians in group practices often can only refer to panels of mental health professionals identified by the patient's MCO, or to the hospital or group where the physician works or has a contract.

A Doctor of Medicine (MD) is not the only medical professional who can make referrals to mental health professionals. There is also the Doctor of Osteopathy (DO) who treats in a holistic manner and considers all body systems as interrelated with an emphasis on the musculoskeletal system. The primary care movement has caused a resurgence in the general practitioner or family doctor. Physicians who develop a personal relationship with their patients and their families may be more open to learning about or referring for mental health issues that impact primary medical care. Approximately 61 percent of DOs and 34 percent of MDs are primary care physicians (PCPs). Until a few years ago, most physicians were in independent practice maintaining professional relationships with hospitals or clinics in their area. In today's marketplace, many other medical professionals can make mental health referrals:

- *Physician Assistant (PA).* PAs practice under the supervision of a licensed D.O. or M.D. There are over 30,000 in the United States, and the field has been identified as one of the faster growing medical professions.
- *Nurse Practitioner (NP).* They work under the supervision of licensed physicians. A Gallup poll shows 86 percent of the public is willing to see a nurse practitioner for everyday healthcare (Wilson, 1996).
- *Nurse-Midwife (CNM).* CNMs must first be a registered nurse, complete a master's program, and take a national exam to become a Certified Nurse-Midwife. They work in hospitals, birth centers, private practices, HMOs, clinics, and more.

From the perspective of the U.S. consumer, there is a wide variety in the kind of medical practitioner patients will have in their first contact unless they are part of an organized health system such as an HMO. Individuals may have their first medical contact in an emergency ward or with the school nurse. Many specialties provide referrals:

Surgeons	Endocrinologists
Ob/Gyn	Psychiatrists
Pediatricians	Neurologists
Gerontologists	Internists
Allergists	Cardiologists
Gastroenterologists	

Your expertise, services, experiences, and products will dictate the kind of medical specialist you can complement most effectively.

The Marketplace

The profile of today's physician is changing. Over 40 percent of medical school admissions are women and many physicians from outside the United States are entering the marketplace. The free-standing independent practice is disappearing, and physicians often take positions with some form of managed care and experiencing a decline in income and autonomy. Physicians are forming group practices in an effort to regain control of their profession. Within MCOs, the gatekeeper primary care physician (PCP) may or may not be knowledgeable about mental health symptoms or issues.

Psychotherapists can help physicians reduce the need for medical services, increase patient satisfaction, and improve treatment compliance. They can also offer new skills to help physicians improve the doctor/patient relationship and increase team performance. We can no longer assume the position of passive recipients of medical professional referrals, but must be proactive in helping physicians solve their professional and personal problems. We recommend you meet them as colleagues who are interested in serving the needs of the community as well as promoting professional success.

Psychotherapists can help physicians reduce the need for medical services, increase patient satisfaction, and improve treatment compliance.

Developing a referral relationship with medical professionals is a long-term project. Physicians can be difficult to meet due to their hectic schedules or can be difficult to talk to personally because of conflicting professional styles. Physicians are outcome oriented and psychotherapists tend to be process oriented. The key to establishing referrals from doctors may be to work your way through the office staff. Often it is the physician support staff who makes the referrals to mental health practitioners after the physician has indicated a need for mental health services. Because physicians and their office staff are very busy people, you need to persevere in your attempts to develop a working relationship. One way to do so is to collaborate with medical professionals in addressing market issues. As the field becomes more computerized, technologized, and mechanized, the human factor is becoming more and more important. As a result, the "human factor" in a client/physician relationship becomes an important market issue.

The key to establishing referrals from doctors may be to work your way through the office staff.

Patient satisfaction is based on personal validation and comfort when a patient meets with his or her doctor. Yet managed care is constantly reducing the time a physician can spend with a patient. Patients do not want to feel like a cog in the medical machine. By providing services for those patients who seek one-on-one human contact, more undivided attention, or special treatment, psychotherapists can be an extension of services offered by physicians.

The role of the mental health professional is to help medical processionals address these issues. Psychotherapists can offer services for the mentally ill and relationship-hungry patients, and human skills and collaborative services for physicians.

Working with Physicians

Your Personal History

Almost everyone has some history with the medical field. Starting as a child and eventually, into adulthood, these experiences have created your feelings and attitudes about the medical profession. As a mental health professional, you may have completed mandatory internships or had jobs working in some kind of medical setting. The experiences you had, good and bad, colored your view of the medical professional. Create a mindmap of your connections to the medical field. Were your experiences negative, positive, or neutral? Whom did you enjoy working with; who was the most helpful? Are there any medical professionals among your friends or their spouses? Try to remember and review each contact you have had. (When you are through, ask yourself if you can honestly work with physicians and feel good about the relationship. Have you been hurt or disappointed? Do you carry any unresolved feelings about the field?)

Niche Experience

If you have a medical background, you are well suited to work with physicians since you already speak their language and may understand their culture. Differences in terminology and professional culture are major obstacles mental health professionals and medical professionals must overcome for successful collaboration. To increase your understanding of the field, consider seeking out a medical professional who will meet with you to discuss crossover issues into the medical field.

Listen to how physicians frame the patient's condition and develop bridges between their framework and yours.

Medical Family Therapy

Today's medical advances have created a situation in which many old and young people live on in spite of illness and medical disabilities (i.e., low birthweight infant survival, brain damage, cancer, Aids treatment and more). In addition to surviving through diseases or disorders once considered "incurable," families are also impacted by lifestyle illnesses such as smoking, eating disorders, and alcohol and drug abuse.

These so-called successes of modern medicine and consequences of unhealthy lifestyle choices have created situations in which families have to deal with the burden of extended treatment. The stress imposed on the family amplifies family problems and can create new pathological systemic responses. Marriage and family therapists are expertly trained to identify and help change these unhealthy system patterns.

Psychotherapists who deal with family systems and are able to collaborate with the medical field, Medical Family Therapists (MFTs) are a resource for these families (McDaniel, Hepworth, & Doherty, 1991). Families need to feel like they have more choices, need help in making decisions, and want support managing their problems. These families need new ways of dealing with loss, grief, family stress, financial problems, contagion, emotional depletion, the psychological aspects of illness and learning how to deal with the personality changes of a loved one with a chronic illness and/or disability.

Families need to feel like they have more choices, need help in making decisions, and want support managing their problems.

MFTs can make extended treatment more humane, more clinically effective, and more cost effective. They can help design changes in the system of delivery of services, interface between the family, patient, and healthcare systems. They can help to improve treatment compliance, reduce failure to thrive reactions, and address overutilization and underutilization of services.

The ecological approach uses multiple perspectives to create entirely new approaches.

Medical family therapists generally use an ecosystemic model. They address the biological, psychological, social, and cultural aspects of the patient's life. They look at interaction patterns, address belief systems, and help manage resources and become an interpreter for the patient and the family about current and future treatment for the family member. The ecological approach "uses multiple perspectives to create entirely new approaches. Providers shift their perspectives from a single discipline to the interfaces between the interdisciplinary systems and the communications between systems" (McDaniel et al., 1992). There is a professional association for this group, the Collaborative Family HealthCare Coalition. Their membership office can be reached at (716) 244-6347. Another resource on integrated delivery systems is *The Keys to Success in Creating Integrated Delivery Systems,* a report developed by the Managed Care Information Center, telephone (800) 333-7771.

Settings

Some primary care physicians, nurse practitioners, and other medical professionals are approaching mental health professionals to become part of an integrated practice.

Some primary care physicians, nurse practitioners, and other medical professionals are approaching mental health professionals to become part of an integrated practice. This requires that the mental health professional be well-known and well thought of in their community in order to be sought out. MFTs might work in primary care settings, nursing homes, and group medical practices in addition to their private practice. Other opportunities are to be on-site consultant, a referral resource, or an off-site consultant. Alternative settings could be any specialty medical setting such as a diabetes center, a rehabilitation-fitness center, a neurology clinic, a children's hospital, or community medical emergency center.

Obstacles to This Niche

For the medical professional and the mental health professional to work together successfully, they must make a concerted effort to dialogue about their differences and find commonalities.

Physicians and psychotherapists can have extreme differences in their models and goals of treatment. Mental health services often come with a stigma attached to them, and the PCP must deal with this reaction when recommending or offering mental health services. For the medical professional and the mental health professional to work together successfully, they must make a concerted effort to dialogue about their differences and find commonalties, such as a desire for the patient's treatment to succeed and an acknowledgment of how their differing skills and gifts enhance one another. They must collaborate on a treatment plan and gain increased knowledge about each other's field.

There are three basic forms of collaboration:

1. *Cotherapy.* This can be done with both professionals meeting the patient and family together, or meeting with them individually in their separate offices. If the consultations are done separately, there must be a system of communication to support collaboration.

2. *Consultation*. Either professional acknowledges the importance of the other's work and consults about the impact of both approaches on the patient's treatment outcome.
3. *Limited Referral*. Varying degrees of communication and collaboration or cooperation between the professionals.

This niche market is for mental health professionals who feel comfortable in the medical arena. They must have a commitment to learning the language, treatment approaches, and medical models of working with a patient. They must be willing to learn how to communicate with medical professionals in a way that promotes understanding of psychotherapeutic treatment approaches and goals.

Physician Services

Psychotherapists can offer physicians many kinds of service, but they fall into two general arenas. The first one includes services that can be offered to patients. Always keep in mind that you have a lot to offer patients of the medical professional. Review the following list and try to add to it:

- Hypnosis.
- Biofeedback.
- Improvement of patient compliance.
- Dealing with chronic illness or fatigue.
- Encouragement of a more rapid recovery due to increased treatment compliance.
- Midlife and aging issues—menopause, empty nest, reduced physical performance.
- Reduction of patient fear and pain.
- Increased patient self-reliance and responsibility.
- Services for disorders related to anxiety, depression, or grief.
- Stress-induced illness relief.
- Behavioral or habit change.
- Lifestyle change.
- Discipline problems in children—parenting skills.

- Family therapy for the families of chronically ill or terminally ill patients.
- Referral source for any other identified psychological issue.

The second arena covers services physicians can use for themselves and their office staff. The following suggestions are in that category. Try to generate more of your own ideas:

- Improvement of communication and goodwill between doctor and patient.
- Teamwork skills and techniques for doctors and their staff.
- Increased patient satisfaction.
- Improved time management.
- Educating the physician about identifying specific mental illnesses such as depression and suggesting screening tools they can use with their patients that can help them make referrals for mental health services (e.g., Beck Depression Inventory).
- Burnout and compassion fatigue.
- Staff team building.
- A referral source to help them deal immediately with psychological problems.

Engaging the Marketplace

Making a Match. Begin by identifying the type of medical professional you are most interested in, and with whom you are likely to build the best relationship. For each professional you identify, create a Physician and Practice Profile, as shown in Figure 3.1.

Competitors

Once you have identified the kind of medical professional you are going to target, look in the Yellow Pages of your local directory to see whether anyone else is offering the services or products you are considering.

Once you have identified the kind of medical professional you are going to target, look in the Yellow Pages of your local directory to see whether anyone else is offering the services or products you are considering. Go to Chamber of Commerce meetings in your area, and network to locate others with similar services or products. When you have identified these people, gather information about their services and products, the fees

Name ____

Specialty ____

Hospital alliances ____

MCO alliances ____

Address ____

Telephone ____

Office hours ____

Mutual contacts ____

____

Mutual interests (seminars, conferences, workshops, conventions) ______________

____

Type of practice or specialty ____

Size of practice ____

Physician's training and background ____

____

Attitude of orientation toward psychotherapy ____

____

Personal interests and involvements ____

Professional contacts and resources ____

Community involvements ____

Publications ____

Most of this information is available in *The Official ABMS Directory of Board Certified Medical Specialties* (Elsevier, 1996).

FIGURE 3.1 Physician and Practice Profile

they charge, the geographic locations they service, and the medical professionals with whom they work.

Many mental health professionals approach physicians for referrals. Try to make your approach as personal as possible and do your research to make certain your contact is appropriate. What you are offering must be relevant to the medical professional that you are approaching. *Stand out from the crowd.*

Strategic Marketing Plan

Since physicians are difficult to reach, another path to make contact with them is to attend continuing education courses they frequent. Contact the organizations that sponsor professional meetings and get on their mailing lists so you can attend other professional gatherings that physicians attend. These include educational opportunities, research projects, and other meetings of medical interest. Contact the departments of local hospitals, universities, and research organizations. Find out what their projects are and see if you can get on a research team in an area such as gerontology, pain control, sleep, pediatric research, depression, or eating disorders. Whatever project or meeting you get involved in, you must show honest interest in the topic or you will be labeled as an opportunist, which will do you more harm than good.

Networking

The best way to network with physicians is by verifying your client's most recent physical or other medical information to confirm your *DSM* diagnosis. Have each client sign a release to contact his or her primary care physician (see Resources, Figure 3.10) and continue with follow-ups as appropriate, including:

The best way to network with physicians is through verifying your client's most recent physical or other medical information to confirm your DSM diagnosis.

- Psychological issues that might impact treatment compliance.
- Psychological issues that are manifesting through medical problems or medical office visits.
- Psychopharmacological consults and follow-ups to medication response and compliance.
- Habit change that contains a medical component.

This networking route is not to be abused. It is, however, the single best way to get to know physicians and other medical professionals who are treating your client.

Attempting to approach physicians when you are not working with any of their patients, can be notoriously difficult. The best entry is through the office manager. Get to know that person first. Ask how you can help, ask about his or her interests, challenges, and the frustrations of managing a medical practice. Offer to help the manager and staff through phone consults or in-house training. Ask for ideas on how you can work with the office he or she manages. Above all, respect the manager's position, which involves dealing with many problems on a daily basis. Be a part of the solution, not another problem.

To meet physicians on off hours, you will need to be where they go when they are not working. Get involved in the chamber of commerce, golf club, yacht club, library board, and school boards. Bring up the topic of "work" in a way that is not intrusive to their free time. Include community and specialty physicians in your Practice Resource Directory (see Chapter 2). As you develop your physician profile, stop by each office and introduce yourself and leave some information about your services. Follow up in a couple of weeks to see if they need any more information. Your informational brochures can be strategically designed for each specialty, (e.g., Pediatricians—Parenting Issues; Internists—Smoking Cessation). Information for your publications on mental health issues can be obtained from the National Institute of Mental Health. Their information is copyright free and may be reproduced or duplicated without permission from the Institute, although we recommend giving them credit for the resource.

Physicians also may gather at workshops for other interests:

- Investment opportunities.
- Practice-building.
- Bill collection.
- Malpractice protection.
- Tax reduction.
- CE vacation opportunities.

Look in medical journals and professional publications for events and check physicians' sites on the Internet. Since a major gathering place for

Contact psychiatric hospitals and walk-in psychiatric services in your area. Include them in your Practice Resource Directory and leave information about your services.

physicians is hospitals, there are many opportunities for physician contact at these sites.

Hospitals

Contact psychiatric hospitals and walk-in psychiatric services in your area. Include them in your Practice Resource Directory and leave information about your services. Look for IPAs (Independent Practice Associations) in your area and do the same. To network more effectively, contact local medical societies and obtain a copy of their directories. Contact the medical director, director of nurses, and the director of outpatient mental health services.

Inquire about hospital privileges or get involved informally when a patient is hospitalized. When your client is discharged, and after obtaining the required releases, write a report about how the hospitalization or hospital services impacted and is being integrated into your overall treatment plan. Send a copy to every physician who was part of the treatment team. Send periodic progress updates until the client discontinues or terminates treatment. This serves a twofold purpose of keeping them informed in case the client requires future hospitalization and keeps the physicians apprised of your clinical professionalism.

Whenever possible, attend clinical staff meetings that relate to any of your clients such as: treatment planning, discharge planning, and team meetings.

When you join any of their meetings, you must know how to understand and speak their language. Don't ramble on about how you have planned your treatment and how it is progressing; be specific and clinically clear and accurate at all times.

When you present or send reports, follow a standard format (Zuckerman, 1997) and make all your clinical notes, if you include them, problem oriented. Any clinical notes should be in a medical format such as SOAP notes—Subjective, Objective, Assessment, and Plan. Or use some other kind of standardized format (Wiger, 1997). Your standard case management procedure should include contact with every client's PCP.

Case Management and Office Procedures

Intake. When you complete a client intake, gather information about their PCP. Obtain a release and send a request for your client's current medical records. Physicians can be impressed with the thoroughness of the attention that you give your clients by considering their medical care in your clinical picture. Typically, clients will already be involved with these physicians: general practitioner, gynecologist/obstetrician, internist, neurologist, pediatrician, and psychiatrist.

Ask about other health professionals the client is currently working with as well. It is good practice to know about any biomedical issue that may impact your work and also provides an opportunity to network with other professionals.

It is good practice to know about any biomedical issue that may impact your work and also provides an opportunity to network with other professionals.

Use a mental status exam for each patient at intake. Write a comprehensive report that includes:

Chief complaint and reason for referral.

Identification—general description of patient.

History of problem.

Current functioning and mental status.

History, psychosocial.

Family history.

Significant traumas.

Psychodynamic constellation.

Relationship history.

Diagnostic impression.

Treatment plan.

DSM-IV protocols.

Goals.

Behavioral plan.

Interventions.

Prognosis/conclusions and recommendations.

This information will help you communicate about your client to medical professionals. Anything you can include in your reports that the physician can do to help their patient should be included.

Offering Nonmedical Seminars and Workshops for Physicians

There are many workshops you can offer that physicians may find valuable. You can create your own workshops or order training packages from training companies. A training resource web site is www.tcm.com/trdev. A few typical workshops are:

- 1001 ways to reward employees.
- How to hire office staff.

- Team building.
- Communication skills for front office staff.

Specialty Promotion

Use the Internet to identify sites that address your specialties.

Use the Internet to identify sites that address your specialties. Many times they link to treatment facilities and providers. Send information about yourself to these locations. For example, if your specialty is eating disorders, you will find a national listing of treatment centers. Many times, these centers are looking for professionals for their clients when the treating physician discharges them. To begin your search, check out the site for the National Institute for Mental Health at www.nimh.nih.gov. The following paragraphs discuss other niche specialties.

Depression. Depression is a high incident, underdiagnosed, and undertreated medically indicated problem. During a Symptom Driven Diagnostic System for Primary Care computer screening of patients, Kaiser Permanente in Oakland, California, found that 20 percent of the patients who answered the questions were diagnosed with a mental disorder, and 46 percent of this group had never been told by their PCP that they had a mental problem ("Practice Advisor," August 1998, *Open Minds*, 5, 8). Host a depression screening in your office. It brings attention to your specialty and serves an honest need. You might network with other professionals who would host a screening in their office.

Adolescents. Work with dermatologists who see teens with skin problems such as acne. Skin problems often affect teens' self-esteem during a time when acceptance by their peers is paramount in their mental health.

Pain Management and Control. Network with internists around presurgery consultations. When presurgery and postsurgery consultation is provided, there are fewer complications, faster recovery, reduced need for medication, and decreased overall stress in relation to surgery events. This lower stress improves the immune system, helping support less complications to this procedure (*Practice Strategies*, November 1998). You can obtain Pain Management Certification from the American Academy of Pain Management at (209) 533-9744 or www.aapainmanage.org.

Obesity. In 1997, the American Heart Association launched a war on fad diets, identifying them as short-term solutions to long-term problems. Offer services to help patients deal with their excess weight in a safe and healthy way supporting long-term weight loss and wellness maintenance. This approach helps create and sustain a healthy self-image, positive attitude, and proper nutrition.

Outreach Vehicles

Letters

There are many reasons to contact a physician. Here are some occasions that could warrant a letter:

- Introducing your practice.
- Offering a video series.
- Offering a new service.
- Holding an open house.
- Announcing community groups that meet in your office.
- Inquiring about a personal physician of some type.
- Having a client in common.
- Starting a new treatment group.
- Responding to a mailing.
- Expressing thanks for a referral.
- Following up a meeting at a social event.
- Forwarding a psychological evaluation or progress report.
- Announcing training in a new technique.

Figures 3.2 through 3.6 show some sample letters you can individualize for your practice. Notice the left side of the letterhead, which includes the organization's mission statement and below that, a list of the topics the niche market may be interested in. Adapt this list to refer to your skills and the specialties you have developed for each niche market you reach out to.

Alpha Centre

6 Pleasant Street Suite 214 Malden MA 02148 617-322-3051

Our mission is to be a professional resource in support of the health and well-being of
- *The whole person*
- *Families*
- *Businesses, institutions, and*
- *Municipalities*

in the service of creating caring community

Our services include psychoeducational workshops on:

EATING DISORDERS

HOW TO CHOOSE THE RIGHT THERAPIST

SELF-ESTEEM AND HEALTH

PARENTING TRAINING

COMMUNICATION SKILLS AND CONFLICT MANAGEMENT

STRESS MANAGEMENT

MEDIATION

BEING A SUCCESSFUL SINGLE

SURVIVING AND THRIVING AS A STEP-FAMILY

FAMILY MEETINGS

MENTAL ILLNESS WHAT IS IT?

SUCCESSFUL AGING

SUCCESSFUL LIFESTYLE CHANGE

Dear __________ :

Mental health services can sometimes be of help to your patients. We want to take this opportunity to advise you of the opening of The Alpha Centre in Malden. We provide counseling for the following medical related conditions:

- Eating Disorders
- Depression
- Post Traumatic Stress Disorders
- Suicide prevention
- Stroke recovery and helping the family support and adjust to change
- Dealing with chronic medical conditions
- Increasing medical treatment compliance
- Adjusting to lifestyle changes due to medical conditions
- Support groups for cancer patients and their families
- Stress reduction
- Adjustment disorders
- Seasonal Adjustment Disorder SAD

We provide plsychoeducational material for you, your staff and your patients. If you would like copies of our informational brochures on any of these topics, please indicate on the enclosed return postcard.

Feel free to contact our office for any information about our practice.

Sincerely,

FIGURE 3.2 Sample Letter of Introduction

Dear _________ :

Video series

The Alpha Centre is offering a free drop-in film series on eating disorders. You and your staff are invited to attend and see how eating disorders are portrayed to the public in film. After each screening we facilitate a topic discussion and answer questions about the many different kinds of eating disorders. We are offering a special screening for professionals and their staff, which we have indicated below. Clinical issues as well as general questions are answered about the psychodynamics of eating disorders after the screening.

A View of Eating Disorders

Date: Friday, June 1 from 3 PM to 5 PM
Location: Alpha Centre

A copy of our informational brochure and newsletter is enclosed. If you would like additional copies for your staff or patients, please indicate on the enclosed return postcard.

Sincerely,

FIGURE 3.3 Sample Letter for a Drop-In Series

Dear ___________ :

The Alpha Centre is holding an open house for all health service professionals in Malden. This is an opportunity for us to network and establish a health service community for our city. Bring information about your professional services and plenty of business cards. You and your office staff are invited to join us.

Information about our centre and sample informational brochures and newsletters are enclosed. Please feel free to contact us about our services.

Sincerely,

FIGURE 3.4 Sample Letter for an Open House

Dear ___________ :

I received a call the other day from an individual in need of counseling who told me it was upon your recommendation. Thank You. I find referrals from colleagues to be the most validating and rewarding.

Please send me information about your current services. I have enclosed some of my business cards in case there are other patients who may benefit from my work.

Thanks again. Please feel free to contact my office for any information about my practice.

Sincerely,

FIGURE 3.5 Sample Thank-You Letter

Dear __________ :

It was a pleasure to meet you at the recent Chamber of Commerce meeting. I want to follow up our informational meeting with a more formal educational contact about my professional services.

I practice at the Alpha Centre, which is wheel chair accessible and close to public transportation. My specialities include eating disorders, stress reduction, and depression. My practice partner is Jean Wright, who specializes in spiritual counseling and mediation. I am licensed as a Marriage, Family therapist, a Mental Health Counselor, and am certified in Group therapy. My clinical experience has been in a variety of mental health settings and currently I am doing research on bingeing, eating disorders, and morbid obesity.

My fees are $125 for individual visits and $45 for groups. Other services such as testing, home visits, and workshops are attached. I rarely turn away clients because of their inability to pay and take most insurances. Currently, I have a group for Binge Eating Disordered patients.

My main focus is the health of the individual and their families. I consider the family as a system that is involved in the health and illness of the individual. If you have any questions or would like to visit my office, please call me at (781) 322-3051.

Sincerely,

FIGURE 3.6 Sample Letter to a Contact Met at a Networking Event

When you send out any outreach piece, include a mail-back card personalized for that professional, as shown in Figure 3.7.

Your practice brochure needs to include the services and products you offer.

Brochures

Professional Practice Brochures. Your practice brochure needs to include the services and products you offer, (e.g., counseling services for individual,

Return Address | Stamp

Alpha Centre
Linda Lawless, Jean Wright
6 Pleasant Street, Ste. 214
Malden, MA 02148

Yes, I received your mailing card

- ☐ Please put me on your mailing list for future events, services and products.
- ☐ I would like more information regarding your services.
- ☐ Please send sample informational brochures

Name ______________________________

Address ______________________________

Telephone ______________________________

Alpha Centre Mission Statement
To be a professional resource in support of the health and well-being of
the whole person
families
business, and institutions, and
municipalities
in the service of creating caring community

FIGURE 3.7 Mail-Back Card

couples, and families). Specify age ranges if you specialize in children or elder populations. Offer groups for your specialties and psychoeducational training opportunities (such as stepparenting and parenting classes). Hold drop-in events that support your specialties. As you schedule events, you have another reason to send information to all the professionals in your community. Figure 3.8 illustrates a professional practice brochure.

Informational Brochures and Newsletters. Informational brochures are also a good way to get your name into the medical professional's office. Be strategic as well as fundamental. The brochure or newsletter format should include:

- An introduction that covers the mission statement of your practice (Ackley, 1997).
- A brief overview of the problem and a listing of sample problems (Figure 3.9).
- Community resources.
- Optional—A simple self-assessment.

Examples of strategic topics for physicians include:

Specialty	*Topic*
Gerontology	Aging gracefully
General Practice	Stress management
OB/Gyn	Menopause
Pediatrician	Parenting

A physician brochure or newsletter could focus on solutions to professional life:

- Patient-professional communication.
- Stress management.
- Dealing with managed care.
- Life balance.
- Burnout.
- Balancing multiple priorities.

The Alpha Centre offers psychoeducation, counseling, consultation and assistance with locating needed resources. We are sensitive to and respectful of personal confidentiality..

Call 781.322.3051 for

Individual Counseling and Personal Growth
By considering interpersonal behaviors in your relationships and work experiences, and gaining awareness of your relational style and goals, new options and resources may be developed.

Family Therapy
By exploring relationship patterns, the family may develop healthier styles of relating and dealing with problems.

Workshop and Retreat Leadership
We will team with you in planning and facilitating a program and process which will be forward you goals for a successful group experience.

Couples Counseling
Couples are assisted in clarifying their hopes and expectations of the relationship, enhancing communication skills, and co-creating the type of relationship they desire.

Separation Counseling and/or Divorce Mediation
When a relationship must end, impartial caring mediation can help you take charge of arrangements, avoid unnecessary injury to spouses and children, and save an average of 90% of the cost of litigated divorce.

Professional Consultation
If you are wondering what to do about a situation and would like an objective viewpoint and/or resources or referrals, we will work with you in reaching your goals.

The Alpha Centre

Sliding Fee Scale available for Uninsured and Private Pay Clients

---

Accessible by Public Transportation (Take the Bus or The Orange Line to Malden Center)

Parking Available On-street and in Parking Garages or Parking Lots

---

Elevator Building
Handicap Accessible

Directions by car to Malden:

Rt. 60 East to Main Street; turn left onto Main Street and take the second left onto Pleasant Street; 6 Pleasant Street is at the corner of Main and Pleasant Street

The Alpha Centre
6 Pleasant St. Ste. 214
Malden MA 02148

Phone: 781.322.5051
Fax: 781.662.8575

It is a sign of wisdom, not weakness, to ask for help.

The Alpha Centre

a resource for medical professionals who are seeking mental health resources for their patients and their practice

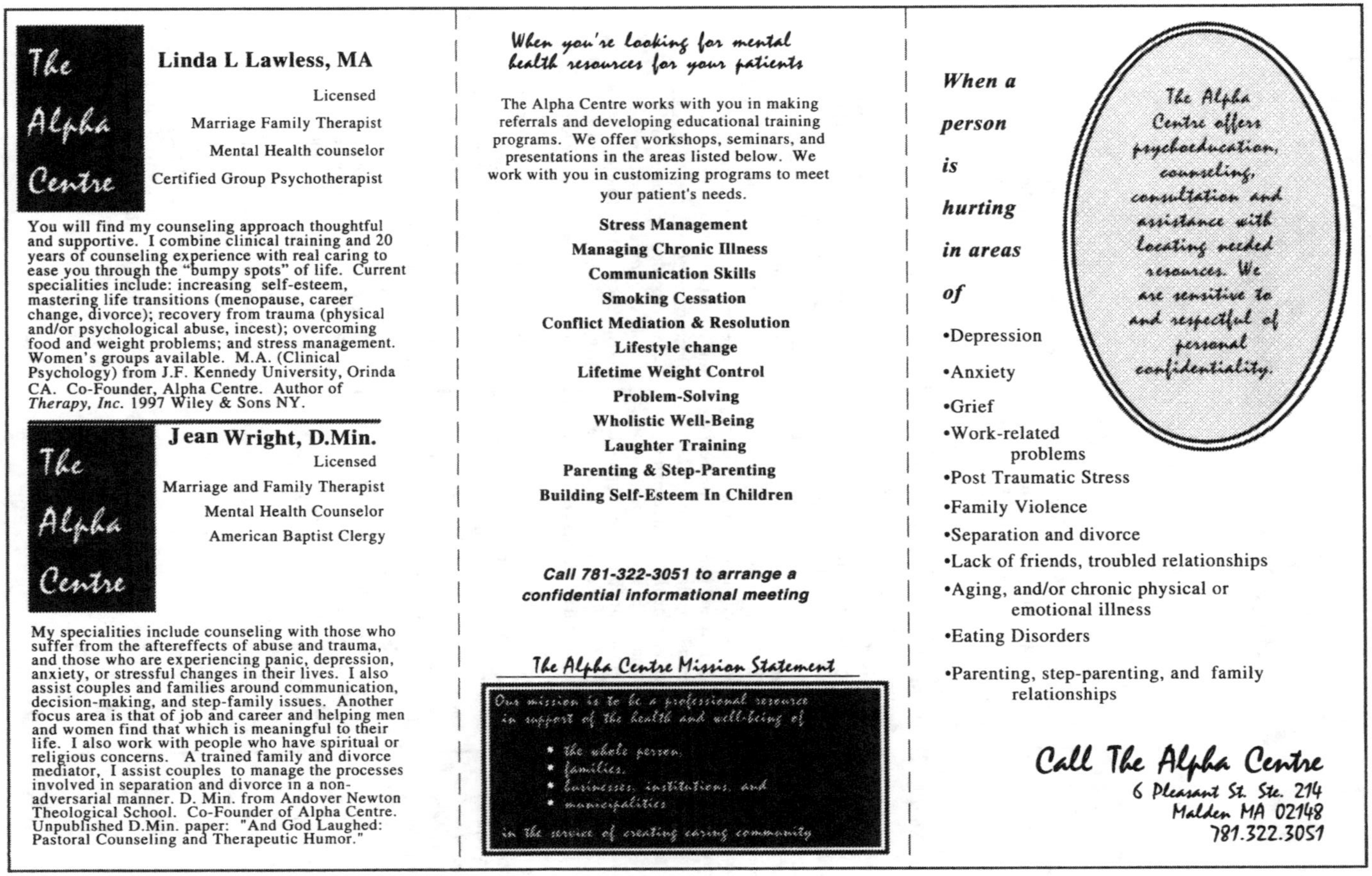

FIGURE 3.8 Professional Practice Brochure

Vol. 1 No. 1 August 18, 1998

The Alpha Centre

6 Pleasant St. Suite 214 • Malden MA 02148

Binge Eating Disorders

This information is offered as a psychoeducation piece for clients, their friends and families. For more copies, or articles on other aspects of mental health contact Linda L. Lawless LMHC LMFT CGP @ A Safe Place To Talk - 781. 662.6026

Each year millions of people in the United States are affected by serious and sometimes life-threatening eating disorders. The vast majority--more than 90 percent--of those afflicted with eating disorders are adolescent and young adult women. One reason that women in this age group are particularly vulnerable to eating disorders is their tendency to go on strict diets to achieve an "ideal" figure. Researchers have found that such stringent dieting can play a key role in triggering eating disorders.

The consequences of eating disorders can be severe. Nevertheless, some people with eating disorders refuse to admit that they have a problem and do not get treatment. Family members and friends can help recognize the problem and encourage the person to seek treatment.

This newsletter provides valuable information to individuals suffering fromeating disorders, and to family members and friends trying to help someone cope with the illness. The publication describes the symptoms of eating disorders, possible causes, treatment options, and how to take the first steps toward recovery.

This disorder is identified by episodes of uncontrolled eating or Binging. Individuals with binge eating disorder feel that they lose control of themselves when eating. They eat large quantities of food and do not stop until they are uncomfortably full. Some major food preferences can be sweet foods, fatty foods or salty foods. Usually, they have more difficulty losing weight and keeping it off than people do with other serious weight problems. Most people with the disorder are obese and have a history of weight fluctuations. Binge eating disorder is found in about 2 percent on the general population--more often in women than men. Recent research shows that binge eating disorder occurs in about 30 percent of people participating in medically supervised weight control programs.

MEDICAL COMPLICATIONS

People with binge eating disorder are usually overweight, so they are prone to the serious medical problems associated with obesity, such as high cholesterol, high blood pressure, and diabetes. Obese individuals also have a higher risk for gallbladder disease, heart disease, and some types of cancer. Research at the National Institute of Mental Health, NIMH, and elsewhere has shown that individuals with binge eating disorder have high rates of co-occurring psychiatric illnesses--especially depression.

CAUSES OF EATING DISORDERS

In trying to understand the causes of eating disorders, scientists have studied the personalities, genetics, environments, and biochemistry of people with these illnesses. As is often the case, the more that is learned, the more complex the roots of eating disorders appear.

<u>Personalities</u>

Most people with eating disorders share certain personality traits: low self-esteem, feelings of helplessness, and a fear of becoming fat. In anorexia, bulimia, and binge eating disorder, eating behaviors seem to develop as a way of handling stress and anxieties.

<u>Genetic and environmental factors</u>

Eating disorders appear to run in families--with female relatives most often affected. This finding suggests that genetic factors may predispose some people to eating disorders; however, other influences--both behavioral and environmental--may also play a role. One recent study found that mothers who are overly concerned about their daughters' weight and physical attractiveness may put the girls at increased risk of developing an eating disorder. In addition, girls with eating disorders often have a mother, father or brothers who are overly critical of their weight.

TREATMENT

Eating disorders are most successfully treated when diagnosed early. Unfortunately, even when family members confront the ill person about his or her behavior, or physicians make a diagnosis, individuals with eating disorders may deny that they

FIGURE 3.9 An Informational Newsletter

2 Ed

August 18, 1998

have a problem.

The longer abnormal eating behaviors persist, the more difficult it is to overcome the disorder and its effects on the body. Sometimes, long-term treatment may be required. Families and friends offering support and encouragement can play an important role in the success of the treatment program.

If an eating disorder is suspected, particularly if it involves weight loss, the first step is a complete physical examination to rule out any other illnesses. Once an eating disorder is diagnosed, the clinician must determine whether the patient is in immediate medical danger and requires hospitalization. While most patients can be treated as outpatients, some need hospital care.

Conditions warranting hospitalization include excessive and rapid weight loss, serious metabolic disturbances, clinical depression or risk of suicide, severe binge eating and purging, or psychosis.

The complex interaction of emotional and physiological problems in eating disorders calls for a comprehensive treatment plan, involving a variety of experts and approaches. Ideally, the treatment team includes an internist, a nutritionist, an individual therapist, and psychopharmacologist, someone who is knowledgeable about psychoactive medications useful in treating these disorders.

To help those with eating disorders deal with their illness and underlying emotional issues, some form of psychotherapy is usually needed. A psychotherapist meets with the patient individually and provides ongoing emotional support, while the patient begins to understand and cope with the illness. Group therapy, in which people share their experiences with others who have similar problems, has been especially helpful.

Use of individual psychotherapy, family therapy, and cognitive-behavioral therapy--a form of psychotherapy that teaches patients how to change abnormal thoughts and behavior--is often the most productive. Cognitive-behavior therapists focus on changing eating behaviors usually by rewarding or modeling wanted behavior. These therapists also help patients work to change the distorted and rigid thinking patterns associated with eating disorders.

NIMH-supported scientists have examined the effectiveness of combining psychotherapy and medications. For patients with binge eating disorder, cognitive-behavioral therapy and antidepressant medications may also prove to be useful. Fluoxetine has also been useful in treating some patients with binge eating disorder. These antidepressants may also treat any co-occurring depression.

The efforts of mental health professionals need to be combined with those of other health professionals to obtain the best treatment. Physicians treat any medical complications, and nutritionists advise on diet and eating regimens. The challenge of treating eating disorders is made more difficult by the metabolic changes associated with them.

HELPING THE PERSON WITH AN EATING DISORDER

Treatment can save the life of someone with an eating disorder. Friends, relatives, teachers, and physicians all play an important role in helping the ill person start and stay with a treatment program. Encouragement, caring, and persistence, as well as information about eating disorders and their dangers, may be needed to convince the ill person to get help, stick with treatment, or try again.

Family members and friends should read as much as possible about eating disorders, so they can help the person with the illness understand his or her problem. Once the person gets help, he or she will continue to need lots of understanding and encouragement to stay in treatment.

It is very important that the focus be on the whole person and their lifestyle changes. Since control is often an issue with eating disorders the patient must be in charge of their treatment options. It is vital that friends and family support all efforts toward affecting change and not focus simply on weight gain or loss.

Simple Self Assessment

- I have recurrent episodes of excessive eating
- After I eat I feel uncomfortable physically and emotionally
- I often eat alone because I am embarrassed about how much I eat
- I eat frequently, when I am not hungry.
- I have low self-esteem
- I often feel out of control in relation to eating
- Family or friends have been critical about my weight

If you answered yes to any of the statements above you may benefit from a consultation with a professional. Contact the Alpha Centre for more information @ 781.322.31051

FOR FURTHER INFORMATION

National Eating Disorder Organization - 445 East Grandille Road - Worthington, OH 43085 - (918) 481-4044

The majority of this information is taken from the NIMH who's work is copyright free.

FIGURE 3.9 *(Continued)*

- How to increase patient compliance with recommended treatment programs.
- Dealing with the difficult patient.

Keep the information to two pages and make it easy to read quickly.

Educational audiotapes are another way for busy professionals and their patients to learn of your services.

Educational Audiotapes. Educational audiotapes are another way for busy professionals and their patients to learn of your services. You can create your own audiotapes or recommend tapes that you use in therapy. Some topics that you may want to teach or discuss on tape might include smoking cessation, weight management, meditation and biofeedback, and grief and loss.

Mailing Lists. Use mailing lists for the physician specialties you are targeting. Send outreach on a quarterly schedule. Check the Yellow Pages and Internet for local physician listings. Many cities include listings of specialties and the physicians who provide services on their municipal web page. Let them know about workshops that may be of particular interest to them.

Always ask if the physician has time to talk with you, and when you are told no, ask if you can speak with them about offering mental health or family resources for their patients.

Telephone Script. Physicians are difficult to reach directly. You will have better luck contacting their practice or office manager. Always ask if the physician has time to talk with you, and when you are told no, ask if you can speak with them about offering mental health or family resources for their patients. Follow-up with a note. The script on pages 91–92 is a guide for directing the conversation.

"To Do" List. Use this activity list as an adjunct to your current personal management system. Setting action due dates facilitate accountability and focuses your time use. The sample shown on page 93 is an example of the action items you need to complete to develop this market niche.

Other Promotional Materials

When you offer continuing education events, trade shows, or attend networking gatherings, you can give away many other promotional materials imprinted with your information. Physicians are accustomed to receiving free promotional materials, so select your items carefully so they capture attention. Typical items include calendars, mugs, rolodex cards, pens, stress cards, and web cards. These items can be costly so distribute them wisely.

Telephone Script

Preparing. The physician office manager you are calling has received your letter and brochures in advance:

- Have a copy of the materials before you.
- Review the Physician and Practice Profile to familiarize yourself with the business you are calling.
- Call when you are feeling refreshed and confident.
- Be prepared to not make contact on the first call. Ask for a good time to call back and leave your contact information.
- Be prepared to listen carefully to the practice manager and try to determine what their needs are.
- Take a deep breath and place the call.

Connecting:

- You reach the receptionist or secretary. Identify yourself and your practice, and ask to speak with the practice or office manager. Tell them that you are responding to the request for information if the mail-back card has been returned. If not, say that you are calling to discuss your mailing with him or her. If you know a person in common, let the receptionist or secretary know who has referred or recommended this physician's practice to you. You will most likely receive a higher priority. If the manager is not available, ask that your call be returned, leaving your telephone number with times you may be reached. If you do not receive a return call within a day or two, do not hesitate to call again. Remember that physician's practices are busy. Create a follow-up note to call again.
- You reach the office or practice manager. Have your script at hand and follow it. Keep your text to one page and remember that the call is about building a relationship. In your first paragraph, you begin building the relationship. Introduce yourself and your business; mention that you are a licensed mental health professional:

  This is ______, of ______. I'm a licensed ______ and have been practicing in (name of community) since ______. (If you know someone who knows the physician, mention the person's name and your relationship to him or her at this time. Also let your referral know that you will be calling the physician's practice.)

(Continued)

Presentation. This makes up the second paragraph and contains your reason for calling:

> Did you receive the letter and brochure I mailed on ______? Do you have questions or comments about it?

- Share why you want to network with this particular physician (your particular specialties that correlate with the physician's areas of expertise, i.e., medical family therapy) and that you believe that you share mutual interests, which can benefit you both.
- Ask how long have they been in practice? How did they become interested in medical family therapy? Be interested and keep your questions specific to the topic.
- Ask whether the physician has worked with mental health professionals before. Mention common ground of the two professions (assisting and building a healthy community). You may also base comments on your mission statement. Invite the office manager's ideas about common ground. Develop some questions to ask the office manager:

  > Who do you make referrals to when there are mental health or family needs?

- Ask if any of the informational brochures you sent would be helpful to patients and would they like some more for their waiting room. Offer yourself as a speaker on a topic of interest to them or their patients. Can he or she be helpful or is there another contact? If so, who is the person to speak with?

Close. The third paragraph brings closure to the telephone meeting. If all has gone well and you feel that there is a like-minded interest, invite the office manager to lunch or ask for an appointment to meet and further discuss how you might assist one another. Make appropriate thank yous and close with a "looking forward to meeting you in person" statement.

Affirming. Give yourself a pat on the back! You're on your way to building a niche market.

Completing. Follow up the telephone call with a thank-you note stating that you appreciate the time taken and that you look forward to the possibility of working together around your common interests. If you have scheduled a luncheon meeting and/or appointment to meet, mention it.

To Do List

- Look in the Yellow Pages under Physicians and select the ones in particular specialties to mail your materials to.
- Check physician web sites for your state and locality.
- Check specialty groups and special interest groups for common ground.
- List the physicians you already know; obtain addresses and telephone numbers (date to call their office for possible referrals to other physicians).
- List names of friends, family, and colleagues who might be able to supply names of physicians (date to call them).
- Prepare mailing to physicians by [date].
- Develop brochure by [date].
- Write cover letters by [date].
- Develop and write enclosures by [date].
- Develop and write newsletter by [date].
- Mail packet by [date].
- Schedule calling date.
- Prepare and review your telephone script and practice aloud.
- Integrate all dates with your Goals Plan.
- Mail thank-you note by [date], for example:

Dear ______:

It was a pleasure to learn about Dr. ______'s practice. I enjoyed speaking with you and appreciated the time you gave me. Because we both work with patients with health problems, it is good to have a resource in the medical field for referrals. I look forward to future contact with you. Please do not hesitate to contact me if you have further questions.

Alpha Centre

Request To Primary Care Physician (PCP) for Release of Information

Send to:

____
Physician's Name

____
Street Address, City, Zip

____
Area Code & Phone Number

Client

____
Name/First Middle Last

____
Client SS# & Birthdate

____
Client Street Address, City, Zip

____
Client Telephone Number

I authorize (PCP) ______________________________ , MD to release medical information that might relate to my mental health and/or substance abuse treatment to:
Linda Lawless LMFT LMHC, my mental health provider at:

Linda Lawless LMFT LMHC
PO Box 350
Melrose MA 02176

____
Client Signature   Date

The above authorization is subject to revocation by the client at any time.
A copy of this authorization is valid.

FIGURE 3.10 Release of Information Form

Summary

As the healthcare marketplace changes, medical professionals are becoming more creative in their practice design. Physicians offer services over the Internet, offer retainer relationships to allied health professionals, and make housecalls. In their search for new ways to survive the industrialization of healthcare, mental health professionals can partner with them in addressing the body and mind of their patients. The only limitations in obtaining medical referrals are your creativity and professional stance. This market niche requires a long-term involvement, so be certain it is where you want to make a commitment.

Resources

Release to Obtain Primary Care Physician Information

Figure 3.10 on page 94 shows a sample release form.

Internet Sites

The following sites are a sampler of the kinds of information you can find on the Internet. Once you have visited a few, expand your search through one of the Internet search engines (e.g., Yahoo!).

Professional

American Academy of Child and Adolescent Psychiatry—www.aacap.org

American Academy of Family Physicians—www.aafp.org

American Medical Association—www.ama-assn.org

American Osteopathic Association—www.am_osteo_assn.org

American Psychiatric Association—www.ama-assn.org/home.htm

Association of State Medical Board Executive Directors—www.docboard.org

The Collaborative Family HealthCare Coalition—(212) 675-2447 or www.CFHcC.org

Regional physician guide sample—www.bostonmagazine.com

Pain Management Certification from the American Academy of Pain Management—(209) 533-9744 or www.aapainmanage.org

Related Information Sites

Administration on Aging—www.aoa.dhhs.gov/

Department of Health & Human Services—www.hhs.gov/

Mental Health Net—A good site to get information for your outreach materials. www.cmhc.com

National Institute of Mental Health—www.nimh.nih.gov/

Priory Lodge Education—This site offers continuing education for Family Medical Practice, Psychiatrists, and General Practitioners. www.priory.com/fam

Training and Development Community Center—www.tcm.com/trdev/

Healthcare-Related Associations and Resources

American Academy of Family Physicians
8880 Ward Parkway
Kansas City, MO 64114

American Academy of Pain Management
13947 Mono Way #A
Sonora, CA 95370

American Academy of Physician Assistants
950 North Washington Street
Alexandria, VA 22314

American Medical Association
515 North State Street
Chicago, IL 60610

American Osteopathic Association Department of Public Relations
142 East Ontario Street
Chicago, IL 60611

Physicians Patient Newsletter
(717) 393-1000

Recommended Reading

Dougherty, W., & MacQran, A. (1999). *Family therapy and family medicine*. New York: Guilford Press.

Elsevier, R. (1996). *The official ABMS directory of board certified medical specialties* (29th ed.). New Providence, NJ: Marquis Who's Who.

Kaku, M. (1997). *Visions: How science will revolutionize the 21st century*. New York: Doubleday.

Kroeger, O., & Thuesen, J.M. (1988). *Type talk—The 16 personality types that determine how we live, love and work*. New York: Dell.

Manisses Communications Group. *The keys to success in creating integrated delivery systems: A special report*. Providence, RI: Behavioral Health Resource Press.

Martin, T. (1983). *How to survive medical school*. New York: Holt, Rinehart & Winston.

Maurer, C., & Sheets, T.E. (Eds.). (1997). *Encyclopedia of associations* (33rd ed.). New York: Gale.

McDaniel, S., Campbell, T., & Seaburn, D. (1990). *Family-oriented primary care*. Heidelberg, Germany: Springer-Verlag.

McDaniel, S.H., Hepworth, J., & Doherty, W.J. (1992). *Medical family therapy: A biopsychosocial approach to families with health problems*. New York: Basic Books.

New York Times. (1998). *A book of record*. New York: NY Times Index.

Open Minds. (1998). Computer screening detects depression. *Practice Advisor*, 5(8), p. 4.

Pekkanen, J. (1988). *M.D. doctors talk about themselves*. New York: Delacorte Press.

Walker, K. (1955). *The story of medicine*. New York: Oxford University Press.

Wilson, R. (1996). *Your career in healthcare*. (Vol Barron's).

Zuckerman, E. (1997). *The clinician's thesaurus* (4th ed.). New York: Guilford Press.

4

Strategies for Getting Referrals from Attorneys

While the American population has grown only 20 percent over these past two decades, the number of attorneys has more than doubled. This means that if you live in a metropolitan area, you will have literally hundreds, if not thousands, of possible referral resources.

To better understand and relate to lawyers, you should learn a little about their background. *Stress Management for Lawyers: How to Increase Personal and Professional Satisfaction in the Law* (Elwork, 1997) is a good resource. Dr. Elwork is both an attorney and a psychologist. His book describes the academic experiences of law students and the effect of their rigorous education. Dr. Elwork also describes the work life of many attorneys in private practice; the material is suggestive for the development of topical workshops for lawyers. The film *The Paper Chase* is about the tribulations of law school and continues to be relevant for describing the stress and competitiveness in that environment. These resources will help you develop empathy and understanding toward members of the legal profession, which will guide you in marketing to lawyers.

Identifying the Marketplace

The American Bar Association identified 985,920 licensed lawyers in the United States as of 1997; 27 percent are female. Identifying your market and researching the field are ways to ensure success in your quest for referrals.

Identifying your market and researching the field are ways to ensure success in your quest for referrals.

A large majority of these attorneys are in private practice. Half of all private practice attorneys are in a solo practice. Group practices cover a wide range in size: small—fewer than 10 lawyers; medium—20 to 50 lawyers; large—50 to 100 lawyers; and megafirms—multicity locations with more than 100 lawyers (Foonberg, 1995). Corporate lawyers generally are employed by business entities.

Private practice for mental health professionals and attorneys has many similarities. Therefore, this chapter focuses on building networks with lawyers in private practice. They, like you, are entrepreneurs trying to develop and sustain a thriving practice. They also are trying to earn a living doing what they love and have committed many years of preparation to their profession. Furthermore, they probably share with you some of the same reasons for going into a private practice. This bond can increase your awareness and create an underlying connection with lawyers that can benefit both parties.

There are two primary branches of law—criminal and civil. Criminal law deals with persons charged with serious offenses that harm others. The community regulates penalties for such deeds; legislative bodies develop statutes defining the crime and the frames for punishment. Civil law deals with damages, restitution, and compensatory actions. Legislative bodies are also often involved in writing statutes and restitutional boundaries regarding civil law. Under each of these categories, numerous specialties and subspecialties exist. As you plan strategies to get referrals from attorneys, choose specialties that best suit your practice and comfort level.

Needs of Attorneys

How can you establish mutually beneficial relationships with attorneys? As in all other cases, you do this by identifying their needs and by being able to fulfill these needs. Law school does little to prepare attorneys for the realities of practicing law (building a practice, interpersonal and practice skills, etc.). According to McCormack (1987), four basic skills that attorneys need and do not learn at most law schools are:

1. *Interviewing*. In the first phase of relating to a client, ascertaining the client's goals and needs, clarifying with the client what can or cannot be done, and gaining the client's business.
2. *Counseling*. Giving appropriate advice based on knowledge of the law applicable to the client's case and particular situation.
3. *Negotiating*. Developing multiple strategies and decision making about the process and outcome of the case (when to be cooperative, when to say "no," when to settle, when to continue).
4. *Drafting*. Writing legal documents and contracts.

Although most therapists have no expertise in drafting legal documents, many mental health professionals have training and experience pertinent to interviewing and counseling. Some mental health professionals even have specialized training in negotiating. If you understand the typical patterns of practicing attorneys, as well as what is not taught at law school and is needed by most attorneys, you can develop several creative ideas for potential workshops.

The Bar Associations of most states have an organization that provides resources and support to legal professionals who are experiencing dysfunction.

The Bar Associations of most states have an organization that provides resources and support to legal professionals who are experiencing dysfunction. It may be called Lawyers Concerned for Lawyers (LCL) or the Lawyer Assistance Program (LAP). Look in the business listings of your phonebook for the organization and telephone number. The American Bar Association has a commission focusing on such programs and has a directory of all LCLs/LAPs in the United States and Canada (see Resources). If you are a seasoned therapist who has expertise in substance abuse and other mental health issues, connecting with LCLs/LAPs will provide another referral resource in building bridges to the legal community.

Competitors

Once you have identified the legal markets that interest you, look in the Yellow Pages of your local directory and see if anyone else is offering your services or products. Attend Chamber of Commerce meetings and locate others who have similar interests and may be working on the same issues (e.g., interview with the LCL or LAP). When you have identified these people/groups, gather information about their services and products. Afterward invite them to complete a Resource Directory form, try to ascertain their interests, and investigate working with them on programs or products.

Making a Match

What is the latest lawyer joke you've heard (or told)? Lawyers are a denigrated profession in American culture. If you want to network with them, you must identify your responses, prejudices, and biases toward the legal profession. Return to and review your family-of-origin genogram and ask yourself the following questions as you take a family legal history (if you don't know, become the family investigator, and seek answers to the questions):

- Are there any attorneys, judges, police officers, prison guards, and so on in the family?
- What has been the family response to those persons and their vocation?
- Has anyone in the family needed to hire an attorney at any time?
- If so, what have they shared about their experience? What was the quality of the experience?
- Has anyone in the family been arrested? Has anyone been imprisoned?
- Do you tell lawyer jokes?
- What is your trust level of lawyers?
- Do you have special training that would correlate with attorneys' needs?

Evaluate your attitudes and make sure you feel comfortable working with attorneys and developing alliances before you continue this chapter.

Niche Experience

Evaluate your training and experience and the types of clients you most often work with. Focus your communication based on this foundation. If you have received training in family and divorce mediation, you may focus your networking with attorneys in family law who specialize in divorce. You could also direct it to attorneys who focus on business law (many small and medium-sized businesses are family businesses). Or if you have a specialty in the area of workers' compensation, you may choose to begin with attorneys who specialize in personal injury law. If your focus is gerontology, you may connect with attorneys who specialize in elder law (often a subcategory of family law); and if you specialize in women's issues—particularly trauma, rape, sexual harassment, or abuse—you may want to network with law firms owned by women who are experienced in representing such cases.

You also have many therapist skills available as a general practitioner.

You also have many therapist skills available as a general practitioner. You can provide lawyers with services for work with people in crisis or trauma; assistance with life transitions—job changes, injuries and illness, separations and divorces, grief and loss; or help with clinical issues such as depression, anxiety, and personality disorders; adolescents and young adult concerns; communication skills training; evaluation and assessment, and interviewing.

Here are two highly specific niche areas you may want to investigate:

1. *The Consultant/Expert Witness for the Court System.* This is a highly specialized niche and pays well. Contact an attorney who specializes in the mental health area and ask for the names of psychological experts they currently use. You may also contact a mental health professional in your area with experience in the field. Interview them to learn how they entered the field and to ascertain what criteria are needed to develop a niche as a consultant/expert witness.

2. *Legal Therapist Counselors.* This is a new and potential growth area with roots in Pittsburgh, Pennsylvania, at Duquesne University. In conjunction with the Legal Therapy Institute, Inc., Duquesne offers a post-masters certification program for legal therapist counselors (LTCs). Ronni Burrows, JD, of Pittsburgh, has an LTC in her firm and believes that many attorneys have so much stress themselves that it is often difficult for them to attend to their clients' emotional needs. Enter the LTC. Burrows describes the relationship as one of a "matrimonial law team." An LTC is "a mental health expert who explains the legal systems to clients and creates the emotional connection that attorneys can't—or won't—make. . . . The goal of this type of service is to assist family law clients during the process of divorce. LTCs help clients prepare for the emotional impact of legal and courtroom proceedings" (Daw, 1997/1998).

There are pros and cons to this relatively new area of collaborative endeavor between mental health professionals and attorneys, most particularly around boundary issues and the ethical standards of mental health groups. Provision 3.6 of the American Association of Marriage and Family Therapists *Code of Ethics* states "Marriage and family therapists do not diagnose, treat, or advise on problems outside the recognized boundaries of their competence" (Daw, 1997/1998, p. 11). For more information regarding LTCs, contact the Legal Therapy Institute, Inc. (see Resources).

Whether you consider yourself a general practitioner or a niche specialist, there are many opportunities for developing products or services for the legal community.

Engaging the Marketplace

Practicing "Due Diligence"

"Due diligence" is legalese for "doing your homework." In legal understanding, it is "reducing exposure if things don't turn out well." Practicing due diligence, rather than taking a shotgun approach to your marketing plan, involves considerable research with three important tools: the Yellow Pages, the Internet, and recommendations about attorneys from people you know. Survey the field and talk with knowledgeable people who can commend attorneys before launching a marketing blitz.

Survey the field and talk with knowledgeable people who can commend attorneys before launching a marketing blitz.

Yellow Pages

The Yellow Pages can be a rich resource as you begin putting together a marketing plan. Most attorneys in private practice are listed, as well as other important contacts you need to know about such as lawyer referral services and state, city, and county bar associations (they also have referral services). Major Yellow Page directories often include, within the alphabetical listing of attorneys, a guide of lawyers arranged by practice specialties, which are numerous. The area of family law alone includes divorce, adoption, mediation or arbitration, domestic abuse, elder or gerontological law, and more. Each of these areas may be listed separately.

The Yellow Pages often also contain a guide of lawyers arranged by location. Not all attorneys will be found in these guides, but they help narrow the field for your marketing program. Make use of both large city as well as local community Yellow Page directories. Lawyer referral services can give you a list of attorneys in your community as well as lawyers in specific specialty areas that would complement your particular areas of expertise. This is an easy way to practice due diligence.

The American Bar Association is accessible by Internet as well as most state bar associations and interest groups within the associations.

The Internet

Those of you who have computers and are online or have access to online resources can find numerous informative web sites. The American Bar Association is accessible by Internet as well as most state bar associations and interest groups within the associations. For example, the Massachusetts Bar web site has links to the Massachusetts Black

Lawyers Association, Lawyers Concerned for Lawyers, The Massachusetts Lesbian and Gay Bar Association, the Women's Bar Association, and Boston Bar Association. Each Internet site lists subcommittees with names and addresses of committee members as well as the addresses and telephone numbers of the Bar group, the association leadership, and referral resources. Resources online tend to be user friendly and responsive (see Resources for online addresses of primary sites). Locate and visit your state bar Internet site, familiarize yourself with its resources, and begin to develop your networking plan with what you learn and are able to use from the site.

Personal Recommendations

Whom do you know in the legal field? Ask these acquaintances to suggest and recommend legal colleagues who are practicing in your areas of interest. Ask your peers and other professional colleagues for names of any attorneys they know or have worked with and would recommend as a potential resource. Ask your friends and neighbors. As you begin to collect leads, ask permission to use the contributor's name in the introductory letter you write to attorneys. When you contact an attorney by telephone, use the name of your referral. Recommendations from a reputable, known source greatly help lay the groundwork for bridge building. Foonberg (1995) strongly emphasizes this point: "Your call or letter will always be given a high priority when you can tell the receptionist, secretary, or lawyer that you were 'recommended' or 'referred' by someone. The lawyer will always take your call, if possible, to avoid offending the person who recommended you."

If you have no recommendations from an individual, name the resource you have used to make contact: Yellow Pages, a referral service, newspaper advertisement. Lawyers will be interested in how you heard of them.

Legal Special Interest Groups

There are listings for particular subgroups within the American Bar Association that you may want to consider such as the Women's Bar Association, Attorneys of Color, and Gay and Lesbian Attorneys.

You will want this type of information for developing a mailing list for your services and products as well as for focusing your interests. The

White Pages also contains listings for numerous social issues, some of which may interest you:

- Lawyers Alliance for Nuclear Arms Control.
- Lawyers Alliance for World Security.
- Lawyers Clearinghouse on Affordable Housing and Homelessness.
- Lawyer's Committee for Civil Rights under the Law.
- National Lawyer's Guild. The National Lawyer's Guild is an organization of ". . . lawyers, law students, legal works, and jailhouse lawyers.in the service of the people, to the end that human rights shall be more sacred than property interests" (from their web site; see Resources).

Networking with a group that has interests similar to yours is another avenue for bridge building. Calling the organization, asking for meeting dates, and requesting a mailing list is the first step. Then survey the list for any names you know and share it with colleagues, friends, or family to see whether they know any attorneys on the list. Begin with those to whom you can provide an introduction by letter or telephone.

Networking with a group that has interests similar to yours is another avenue for bridge building.

American Bar Association Groupings

The American Bar Association (ABA) lists the following specialties. Committees represent the various categories and many local bar associations follow the ABA committee pattern. Reviewing this list will help you select those areas of law with which your practice may have an affinity (Foonberg, 1995):

Administrative Law
Administrative and Regulatory Law
Admiralty and Maritime Law
Affordable Housing and Community Development Law
Agricultural Law
Air and Space Law
Antitrust Law
Appellate Judges
Appellate Practice
Arbitration/Mediation
Aviation and Space Technology
Bankruptcy/Insolvency/Reorganization
Business Law

Civil Rights
Communications Law
Constitutional Law
Construction Law
Corporation Law—Banking and Savings
Corporation Law—General Corporate Practice
Corporation Law—Finance and Securities
Corporation Law—In-House Counsel
Criminal Law—Prosecution
Employee Benefits
Entertainment and Sports Law
Environmental Law
Family Law
Federal Trial Judges
Franchise Law
General Practice
Government—Federal Level
Government—State/Local/Urban
Individual Rights and Responsibilities
Insurance Law
Intellectual Property Law
International Law
Labor and Employment
Law Practice Management
Legal Education
Libel
Litigation—Commercial
Litigation—General Civil
Military Law
Natural Resources Law
Patent Law
Private Defense
Product Liability Law
Prosecution (State and Local)
Public Contract Law
Public Utility Regulated Industry
Real Estate Law
Science, Engineering, and Technology
Special Court Judges
State Trial Judges
Taxation—Corporation and Business
Tort and Personal Injury Law
Trade and Professional Associations
Transportation Law
Trust Probate and Estate Plan

Not all the committees have to do with legal specialties, but most of them do. The state and local bar associations will often have committees in the preceding categories and you can ask for a list of attorneys on the committees with which you have the closest affinity. The attorneys in your locality would be an excellent place to begin your due diligence marketing plan since they likely are perceived as leaders in their professional community.

Another important directory is the *Martindale-Hubbell International Law Directory*, which can be found in most law school libraries, government libraries, and many public libraries. The directory provides a free listing for lawyers who want to be included and rates lawyers according to their reputation in the communities (also available on the Internet, see Resources).

The Marketing Plan

After you have scouted the legal field, develop a mindmap that graphically presents the due diligence information streams and areas for building bridges, reflecting your particular areas of interest and specialties.

Your mindmap is an important guide to direct your next phase, which is the developing of Goal-Setting Worksheets, as described in Chapter 2.

Services and Products

Review the section "Needs of Attorneys" to begin to develop services and products for attorneys. Several suggestions for services, such as the following, probably emerged from those needs and could be offered in your office or other community settings. These could also be potential topics for workshops at continuing legal education events:

- Communication skills:
  - Active listening.
  - Reading body language.
  - Emotional cues.
- Stress management (breathing, meditation, time management, movement, guided imaging, establishing boundaries, etc.).
- Dealing with difficult clients (personality disorders, grief and loss issues, etc.).
- Effective interviewing techniques.

- Mediation skills training.
- Families in transition—Divorce and remarriage issues.
- Preventing burnout in the legal profession.
- Issues related to attorney identity formation.
- Establishing your law practice.
- Dynamics of dysfunctional systems (families, organizations, institutions, businesses, etc.).
- Other—your ideas arising from the preceding suggestions or knowledge you have of the legal field.

Continuing Education Programs

Developing workshops or presentations for continuing legal education programs is a particularly efficacious way to build networks. Attorneys most often are in a receptive mode when they are out of the office and at continuing legal education events. Each bar association will have a continuing education committee. Contact the chair and ask to be added to the mailing list. Inquire about the programs they've had over the past one or two years, what the attendance has been, the procedures for developing and offering a continuing education event, how much lead time is required, and so on. Share your areas of interest and specialty and ascertain if any events have focused on those areas. It would also be helpful for you to colead a workshop or presentation with an attorney. This would offer even greater potential for marketing your product/service.

Each bar association will have a continuing education committee. Contact the chair and ask to be added to the mailing list.

Coleading Workshops with an Attorney

Dessa Rosman Stone, PhD, and Henry Gornbein, Esq. provide a prime example of coleading workshops. They have been working together for several years in the area of divorce issues. They also can be part of a mutual referral system. They consider issues of divorce from a multidisciplinary approach. In 1995, they cocreated the Divorce Online web site which receives over 1,300 visitors and over 7,000 hits daily (see Resources). The site carries a national list of professionals (paid advertising), many excellent articles related to divorce and divorce mediation—legal, psychological, real estate, financial, and other aspects of divorce (they can be downloaded free of charge). They also are developing a recommended book list, which will be carried with a link to Amazon.com (see Resources).

Finding Like-Minded Attorneys

Doing the networking described throughout this chapter will likely uncover relationship possibilities for you. Explore the like-interests/like-mindedness and develop a program or product together that could be offered to the legal, therapeutic, and/or local communities, depending on the shaping of the workshop. The following ideas are examples:

Explore the like-interests/like-mindedness and develop a program or product together that could be offered to the legal, therapeutic, and/or local communities, depending on the shaping of the workshop.

- A workshop led by an attorney and a therapist could be developed for the legal community focusing on the psychological aspects of divorce and their implications for the attorney/client relationship.
- For the therapeutic community (including mental health professionals, clergy, physicians, etc.), a workshop could focus on the legal and psychological aspects of divorce; legal issues regarding elders, and so on.
- For the community, such a workshop could focus on legal and psychological aspects of divorce, elder law and issues of aging, the juvenile system and parenting issues, and so on.

Develop a Mutual Referral System with Attorneys

Your clients may need professional advice in an area where you lack expertise; legal consultations and legal services generally fall in this category. As you build relationships with attorneys, you may also use them as a referral resource. Clients appreciate receiving recommendations, but you need to provide more than one name. Referring to attorneys may well result in your beginning to receive referrals from them. This could also lead to coleading workshops with an attorney. Use the Resource Directory Worksheet as a tool to begin networking with attorneys (see Figure 4.1). You should include it with your initial mailing to selected attorneys.

The Alpha Centre

Attorneys Resource Directory Worksheet

Date: ______________________ New: _____ Revision: _____

Name: ______________________

Address: ______________________

Firm: ______________________

Telephone(s): ______________________

Fax: ______________ E-mail: ______________ Web site: ______________

Office Hours: ______________________

Type of Legal Practice: ______________________

Specialities: ______________________

Year Graduated Law School: ________ Law School: ______________________

Languages Spoken: ______________________

Fees: Indicate if you use a sliding fee scale or other forms of payment options (e.g., credit cards, payment plans): ______________________

What else is important that we know about you or your practice? ______________________

____

Thank you for completing this Resource Directory Form.
Return to:
Alpha Centre
6 Pleasant Street, Suite 214
Malden, MA 02148

If you have any questions, please call: The *Alpha Centre* @ 781.322.3051
Linda Lawless, M.A., LMFT/LMHC; Jean Wright, D.Min., LMFT/LMHC

Application Sent Date: ___________ Approved Date: ___________ Follow-Up Date: ___________

FIGURE 4.1 Attorneys Resource Directory Worksheet

Bar Association Meetings

This is a possible way to network with attorneys since they often are receptive to new resources at these meetings:

- Contact your local and state bar associations for dates of their annual meetings and to arrange to rent a booth or table.
- Have items for display and distribution (include any products or services that would be pertinent to the legal community).

  Brochures. In addition to your basic brochures, create flyers highlighting your niche areas and workshop dates. You may also use a brochure describing your particular field, such as marriage and family therapy. These can often be obtained in bulk through your professional association. Be sure to include your name, address, and telephone number on the brochure.

  Business card. Hand out your business card and inexpensive gifts imprinted with your name, office address, and telephone number (writing pens, notepads).

  Sign-in sheet. Allow spaces for name, address, and telephone number. Follow up with a letter thanking them for stopping by your booth.

Outreach Vehicles

You may want to use all the vehicles presented here, develop some of them, or design others better suited to your needs. Allow enough time to create and produce your materials, and use a professional printing service unless you have high-quality computer software. Attorneys set high standards for themselves; they will judge you the same way. Your materials represent you; they will be the basis for the recipients' first impression of you and your practice.

Attorneys set high standards for themselves; they will judge you the same way.

Resource Directory Worksheet (Lawless, 1997). The Resource Directory Worksheet (see Figure 4.1) is a tool to help you connect with attorneys as well as a practice resource for you and your clients. Include a copy of the worksheet with your outreach materials. When attorneys return the worksheet, follow up with an office visit so you can get to know one another better.

The Alpha Centre offers psychoeducation, counseling, consultation and assistance with locating needed resources. We are sensitive to and respectful of personal confidentiality..

Call 781.322.3051 for

Separation Counseling and/or Divorce Mediation
When a relationship must end, impartial caring mediation can help you take charge of arrangements, avoid unnecessary injury to spouses and children, and save an average of 90% of the cost of litigated divorce.

Professional Consultation
If you are wondering what to do about a situation and would like an objective viewpoint and/or resources or referrals, we will work with you in reaching your goals.

Family Therapy
By exploring relationship patterns, the family may develop healthier styles of relating and dealing with problems.

Couples Counseling
Couples are assisted in clarifying their hopes and expectations of the relationship, enhancing communication skills, and co-creating the type of relationship they desire.

Individual Counseling and Personal Growth
By considering interpersonal behaviors in your relationships and work experiences, and goals, new options and resources may be developed.

The Alpha Centre

Sliding Fee Scale available for Uninsured and Private Pay Clients

Accessible by Public Transportation (Take the Bus or The Orange Line to Malden Center)

Parking Available On-street and in Parking Garages or Parking Lots

Elevator Building
Handicap Accessible

Directions by car to Malden:

Rt. 60 East to Main Street; turn left onto Main Street and take the second left onto Pleasant Street; 6 Pleasant Street is at the corner of Main and Pleasant Street

The Alpha Centre
6 Pleasant St. #. 214
Malden MA 02148

Phone: 781.322.5051
Fax: 781.662.8575

It is a sign of wisdom, not weakness, to ask for help.

The Alpha Centre

For when you're seeking mental health support with the personal issues of your clients and are looking for attitudes sensitive to and respectful of legal and confidentiality issues

The Alpha Centre

Linda L Lawless, MA

Licensed
Marriage Family Therapist
Mental Health counselor
Certified Group Psychotherapist

You will find my counseling approach thoughtful and supportive. I combine clinical training and 20 years of counseling experience with real caring to ease you through the "bumpy spots" of life. Current specialties include: increasing self-esteem, mastering life transitions (menopause, career change, divorce); recovery from trauma (physical and/or psychological abuse, incest); overcoming food and weight problems; and stress management. Women's groups available. M.A. (Clinical Psychology) from J.F. Kennedy University, Orinda, CA. Co-founder, Alpha Centre. Author of Therapy, Inc. 1997 Wiley & Sons NY.

The Alpha Centre

Jean Wright, D.Min.

Licensed
Marriage and Family Therapist
Mental Health Counselor
American Baptist Clergy

My specialties include counseling with those who suffer from the after effects of abuse and trauma, and those who are experiencing panic, depression, anxiety, or stressful changes in their lives. I also assist couples and families around communication, decision-making, and step-family issues. Another focus area is that of job and career and helping men and women find that which is meaningful to their life. I also work with people who have spiritual or religious concerns. A trained family and divorce mediator, I assist couples to manage the processes involved in separation and divorce in a non-adversarial manner. D. Min. from Andover Newton Theological School. Co-founder of Alpha Centre. Unpublished D. Min. paper; "And God Laughed: Pastoral Counseling and Therapeutic Humor."

8 Reasons for Divorce Mediation

Divorce mediation spares unnecessary suffering for men, women and children by:

1. Encouraging two-way communication and mutuality;

2. Helping the partners to take responsibility for their own future, and making it as amicable as possible;

3. Substituting practices of fairness, equitability, and cooperation for the usual patterns of concealment, combat, and injury;

4. Shielding children of the marriage from the traumatic effects of observing their parents fight, by taking the needs of all family members into account;

5. Speeding disclosure of assets and negotiated division of property;

6. Facilitating long-lasting agreements around custody, child support, and espousal support;

7. Saving an average 90% of the cost of a contested divorce;

8. Setting a model for resolution of future conflicts.

The AlphaCentre Mission Statement

Our mission is to be a professional resource in support of the health and well-being of

- the whole person,
- families,
- businesses, institutions, and
- municipalities

in the service of creating caring community

When a person is hurting in areas of

- Addiction
- Anxiety
- Grief
- Work-related problems
- Post Traumatic Stress
- Family Violence
- Separation and divorce
- Lack of friends, troubled relationships
- Aging, and/or chronic physical or emotional illness
- Eating Disorders
- Parenting, step-parenting, and family relationships

The Alpha Centre offers psychoeducation, counseling, consultation and assistance with locating needed resources. We are sensitive to and respectful of personal confidentiality.

Call The Alpha Centre
6 Pleasant St. Ste. 214
Malden MA 02148
781.322.3051

FIGURE 4.2 Sample Brochure for Attorneys Specializing in Family and Divorce Law

Advertisement for Bar Association Newsletter. Call the local bar association and ask to speak to the newsletter editor about placing an ad. This form of advertising is often inexpensive.

Brochures. Develop a basic brochure for the legal community that you can then adapt to address your niche or specialty areas. On the brochure shown in Figure 4.2 on pages 112–113, all panels are applicable to any legal practice except the inside middle one, which addresses the specialty of divorce mediation. To highlight another practice specialty, the therapist would simply rewrite that panel:

- A therapist who works with adolescents and/or troubled youth could describe his or her areas of expertise in the niche panel and send the brochure to criminal attorneys as well as attorneys who practice family law, juvenile law, and so on.
- For therapists with experience in substance abuse issues and treatment, the panel would reflect that background and would be appropriate to send not only to attorneys in family law but also to criminal lawyers since substance abuse is often a concomitant of crimes.

Always list your credentials and educational degrees.

Always list your credentials and educational degrees. In an informal survey of attorneys, appropriate credentialing was the topmost characteristic named in seeking referrals for a client.

Since the education of other professional groups regarding the mental health field is always a part of networking, you may want to include a brochure describing your particular field. For example, the American Association of Marriage and Family Therapists has a printed brochure describing Marriage and Family Therapy.

Invite the attorney to complete and return the Resource Directory Worksheet that you enclose with the letter.

Letters. Most attorneys are logical, analytical, fast thinkers and have a great deal of reading to do. They receive large quantities of mail. You want your letters to be clear, concise, and to the point. They need to be easily scanned for content. Keep all correspondence to a single page. Name your referral source and niche specialty. Invite the attorney to complete and return the Resource Directory Worksheet that you enclose with the letter. Figures 4.3 through 4.5 provide sample letters for three situations.

Mail-Back Card. Communication needs to be two-way. Whenever you create a mailing, encourage a response. Including a mail-back card is one way to do this. You may also invite a telephone call from recipients with questions or comments.

Alpha Centre

6 Pleasant Street Suite 214 Malden MA 02148 617-322-305 1

Our mission is to be a professional resource in support of the health and well-being of
- *The whole person*
- *Families*
- *Businesses, institutions, and*
- *Municipalities*

in the service of creating caring community

Our services include psychoeducational workshops on:

Divorce Mediation

Communication Skills

Conflict Management

Stress Management

Being a Successful Single

Surviving and Thriving as a Step-Family

Family Meetings

Mental Illness What is it?

Successful Aging

Successful LifeStyle Change

Relationship Enhancement

How to Choose a Therapist

Dear ___________ :

It was a pleasure to meet you at the Middlesex Bar Association Annual Meeting. Thank you for stopping by our booth. We are actively seeking to build a network with attorneys in Middlesex County who practice in the area of family law and divorce and look forward to having you as part of our referral network. Although we have your card, would you please complete the enclosed Resource Sheet and return to us for inclusion in our resource file.

We believe that we can be of mutual assistance, support, and a resource to one another's practices as we each seek to enhance the well-being of our respective clients.

The enclosed brochure describes services of the Alpha Centre, including Family and Divorce Mediation. We can help your clients with some of the emotional turmoil involved during important life transitions, thereby making your work more enjoyable.

Possessing several years of counseling experience, we opened our Malden office in April, 1997. We are licensed therapists and available for consultation and speaking engagements regarding emotional and/or mental health issues.

We look forward to working together with you on behalf of our shared community life.

Sincerely,

FIGURE 4.3 Sample Letter to Attorney Met at a Networking Event

Dear __________ :

On March 15, 1999, I will facilitate a 3-hour seminar on "Post-Divorce Life Issues". Enclosed is a flyer describing the seminar. Would you please share it with any of your clients who are facing this issue? I am a licensed marriage and family therapist with several years experience in life transitions, step-family issues and family and divorce mediation.

On March 30, I will begin a 6-week support group focusing on step-family issues and challenges. A flyer is enclosed which describes this opportunity. I would appreciate your sharing it with clients whom you believe would benefit from such a group (limited to 7 participants).

The enclosed brochure describes services of the Alpha Centre, including Family and Divorce Mediation. We are also experienced in relationship counseling and family issues. We can help your clients with some of the emotional turmoil involved during important life transitions, therby making your work more enjoyable.

We invite you tobecome part of our Legal Resource Directory be completing the enclosed Attorney Resource Form and returning it to us.

If you wish further information about the groups or our services, please contact me at: (781) 322-3051.

Sincerely,

FIGURE 4.4 Sample Letter to Announce Start-Up of a New Group or Presentation of a Seminar

Dear ________:

Your name was given to us by the Middlesex County Bar Association as the contact person for those who would like to present workshops or seminars as part of your continuing legal education program.

We are experienced workshop and seminar presenters and would like to discuss with you topics we are able to offer the legal community. We can also develop with you a topic of interest.

A sampling of topics we have to offer include the following:

How to Interview a Potential Client
Handling Difficult Clients
Stages of Grief - Death and Loss
Honing Your Listening Skills
Stress Management for Attorneys
Communication Skills

The enclosed brochure describes services of the Alpha Centre, including Family and Divorce Mediation. We are experienced in divorce mediation, relationships and family issues.

Possessing several years of counseling experience, we opened our Malden office in April, 1997. We look forward to meeting with you and discussing our mutual interests.

Sincerely,

FIGURE 4.5 Sample Letter to Legal Continuing Education Committee

Alpha Centre

June 1998
Volume 1, Issue 1

Inside this Issue

Alpha Centre
6 Pleasant St., Ste. 214
Malden, MA 02148
Telephone 781.322.3051

A Community Resource

Linda L Lawless LMFT LMHC CGP
Jean Wright, DMin., LMFT LMHC

What is a caring community? Our vision of a caring community is one in which individuals, families, businesses, institutions, and municipalities put the welfare of the person before profit or power. We can only begin one step at a time and we have begun with ourselves. We invite others to engage in a dialogue about how we can all put people first.

An example at the Alpha Centre is our referral service directories. When someone calls looking for a mental health professional, if we cannot provide the services needed we use a therapist finder to locate someone who may be of help at the closest geographic location possible? We are developing directories for other professionals such as medical, legal, clergy, etc. We invite you to use our referral service. From the 978 or 781 area code, call 1-800-THERAPIST. From other area codes call 781.211.3051. Leave your name, number, and reason for your call and someone will return your call promptly. As a public service this issue of our newsletter focuses on Grief and Loss. If you would like more copies, contact us at 781.322.3051.

Dynamics of Grief & Loss

Jean Wright, D.Min., LMFT LMHC

Clients who seek you out for assistance with legal issues often are confronted with some form of major loss or life transition, i.e., divorce, illness, loss of spouse, child, job loss, or accident.

The emotional dynamics constellated by such life changes will impinge upon the lawyer/client relationship with them and it's outcome. Having some understanding of primary emotional patterns involved will assist your building a helpful relationship with your client/s.

The emotional resolution of a major loss can take 3-5 years depending upon the number of years the relationship lasted and the manner of the loss. A traumatic loss is more complicated than an expected one.

Recognized psychological aspects of the grief process first described by Elizabeth Kubler-Ross are 5 and include:

1) Denial and isolation: The person feels shock and the "it cannot be true" feeling. Denial protects from emotional overload.

2) Anger: "Why me? questions are in the forefront and feelings of anger and blame are projected outward (and inward, often resulting in depression) onto the circle of relationships, including God. Be prepared.

FIGURE 4.6 Newsletter

June 1998

3) Bargaining: The individual may try to rebuild a broken relationship or have fantasies of the same. He/she may stall for time, etc. "If I'm good maybe all will change." They are vulnerable and may be susceptible to saying "yes" to that not in their own best interests.

4) Depression: One of two forms of depression manifest, they are: a mourning related to what has been lost – reactive depression – or a mourning about what is about to be lost – preparatory depression.

5) Acceptance: He/she comes to terms with the inevitability of what has happened and begins to withdraw the investment in what has been lost, turns inward, and if a healthy grief process has evolved, begins to reinvest energies in other directions.

While a woman or man may be struggling with the processes of the ending of a way of identifying oneself, i.e., wife/husband; President of ABC Corp.; "healthy as a horse, etc. as described in the 5 elements above, conjoint with or following along are what have been described as the 5 stages of bereavement (Parkes, 1971)

1) Alarm: a reflexive and physiologic change (increase in blood pressure and heart rate) that occurs when acute stress is experienced.

2) Numbness: an adaptive defense mechanism that protects against being overwhelmed by painful information or experiences.

3) Pining (searching): seeking that which is lost and characterized by hallucinations or pseudohallucinations of the lost, i.e., "I heard him/her calling me."

4) Depression: Despair and disorganization occur, as the loss becomes more real. Memory and concentration are effected. Feelings that one's life now has no meaning are common.

5) Recovery: He/she is able to relinquish what has been and can now turn toward other goals and persons.

Significant Emotions Involved

1) Anger: resentment toward fates, God, self, other/s frustration.

2) Guilt: "Could I have done more?" to prevent the situation; love/hate feelings; survivor guilt.

3) Shame: Feelings of "I'm not worthy, deserving.... something is wrong with me.": Desire to hide out, isolate self.

4) Fear: Facing a forever after changed reality without support of the lost one/s; realization of life's exigencies; overwhelming emotions, "Am I going insane?" The bereaved person (identification) may assume traits of the lost one; a normal process.

5) Sadness/Sense of Loss: Normatively may last 6-18 months.

Signs of Pathologic Grief

Two types of unresolved grief:

1) Delayed or denied: The onset of grieving occurs more than a few weeks after the loss or trauma.

2) Prolonged and unresolved grief: In either of the two types, the following may be symptoms: a) self-reproach or exaggerated guilt; b) over-identification with the lost person; c) fears and phobias; d) frequent physical complaints and no diagnosis of medical problems; e) psychosis; f) substance abuse; g) unable to assume relatively normal activities within a year of the event.

Suggestions for You

1) Be aware of the stages of grief and mourning your clients may be experiencing.

2) In your time with them, ask about losses in their life. If unresolved, emotions pile up and show up.

3) Acknowledge the emotions as normal.

4) Be confident, precise, and specific in verbal and written communications. Memory and concentration are effected by depression and mourning.

5) Be patient. Calls may not be returned. Appointments may be missed/rescheduled. A telephone reminder can be helpful.

6) Refer clients to mental health professionals.

Article adapted from Death & Bereavement by Ginger, C.M., and Dennis P. Review of General Psychiatry. 1988 Goldman, H. H. Ed. For Further Reading: Kubler-Ross, E. on Death and Dying. MacMillan, 1969 – Rice, Joy K., Ph.D. & Rice, David G., Ph.D. (1986). Living Through Divorce. NY: The Guilford Press.

2

FIGURE 4.6 *(Continued)*

Telephone Script

Preparing. The attorney you are calling has received your letter and brochures in advance:

- Have a copy of the materials before you.
- Review your family-of-origin genogram and therapy family diagram as it relates to any relationships in the legal community and be comfortable with the relationships.
- Call when you are feeling refreshed and confident.
- Be prepared not to make contact on the first call.
- Be prepared to focus and take charge of the call since attorneys are busy professionals.
- Take a deep breath and place the call.

Connecting:

- You reach the receptionist or secretary. Identify yourself and your practice, and ask to speak with Mr./Mrs. _____ (attorney). If the mail-back card has been returned, share that you are responding to his or her request for information. If not, say that you are calling to discuss your mailing with him or her. If you know a person in common, let the receptionist or secretary know who has referred or recommended Attorney _____ to you. You will most likely receive a higher priority. If the attorney is not available, ask that your call be returned, leaving your telephone number with times you may be reached. If you do not receive a return call within a day or two, do not hesitate to call again. Remember that attorneys are busy professionals. Create a follow-up note to call again.
- You reach the attorney. Have your script at hand and follow it. Keep your text to one page and remember that the call is about building a relationship. In your first paragraph, you begin building the relationship. Introduce yourself and your business; mention that you are a licensed mental health professional:

  This is ______, of ______. I'm a licensed ______ and have been located in (name of community) since ______. [If you know someone who knows the attorney, mention the person's name and your relationship at this time. Also let your referral know that you will be calling the attorney.]

Presentation. This makes up the second paragraph and contains your reason for calling:

> Did you receive the letter and brochure I mailed on ______? Do you have questions, comments about it? Share why you want to network with ______ attorneys [your particular specialties that correlate with the attorney's areas of expertise] and that you believe that you share mutual interests, which can benefit you both.

- Ask the attorney some questions about his or her development of the interest or specialty. This will help building bridges of trust and openness. Be interested and keep your questions specific to the topic.
- Ask whether the attorney has worked with mental health professionals before. Mention common ground of the two professions (assisting and building a healthy community). You may also base comments on your mission statement. For example, in discussing divorce mediation, include comments about your training and experience in the field. Share that you respect legal and confidentiality issues.
- Ask if there is a regular monthly meeting of the local or county attorneys to which you might come as a guest. If so, to whom should you speak about the possibility of attending? Offer yourself as a speaker on a topic of interest to them. Can the attorney be helpful or is there another contact? If so, who is the contact person?

Close. The third paragraph brings closure to the telephone meeting. If all has gone well and you feel that there is a like-minded interest, invite the attorney to lunch or ask for an appointment to meet and further discuss how you might assist one another. Make appropriate thank yous and close with a "looking forward to meeting you in person" statement.

Affirming. Give yourself a pat on the back! You're on your way to building a niche market.

Completing. Follow up the telephone call with a thank-you note saying that you appreciate the time taken and that you look forward to the possibility of working together around your common interests. If you have scheduled a luncheon meeting and/or appointment to meet, mention it.

Newsletter. Developing a newsletter for the particular professional group/s with which you wish to network is another helpful way to gain name recognition and grow your practice. Depending on the time you have, it can be monthly or quarterly. Your feature article needs to be informative and interesting to readers. In Figure 4.6 on pages 118–119, the newsletter is directed toward family law attorneys.

Telephone Script. Attorneys have exceedingly busy schedules and are likely to experience nonbusiness calls as extraneous and time-consuming. If you choose to call and introduce yourself or respond to material you have received from an attorney, keep the call focused, precise, and brief. Follow up with a note. The script shown on pages 120–121 is a guide for directing the conversation.

"To Do" List. Using several methods to maintain accountability with your marketing and outreach vehicles is helpful for the accomplishment of your networking plan. A simple "to do" list will focus your time and budgeting.

To Do List

- Look in the Yellow Pages under Attorneys and select the ones to receive your mailers.
- Check attorney web sites for your state and locality.
- Check specialty groups and special interest groups for common ground.
- List the attorneys you already know; obtain addresses and telephone numbers (date to call them for possible referrals to other attorneys).
- List names of friends, family, and colleagues who might be able to supply names of attorneys [date to call them].
- Call either the county or state bar associations, for a listing of attorneys in the communities you serve [date to call].
- Prepare mailing to attorneys by [date].
- Develop brochure by [date].
- Write cover letters by [date].
- Develop and write enclosures by [date].
- Develop and write newsletter by [date].
- Mail packet by [date].
- Set calendar calling date.
- Review telephone script and practice aloud.
- Integrate all dates with your Goals Plan.
- Mail thank-you note by [date], for example:

Dear ______:

It was a pleasure to learn of your interest and experience in the field of family law. I enjoyed speaking with you and appreciated the time you spent in our discussion. As we both work with men and women in difficult situations, it is good to have a resource in the legal field for referrals. I look forward to future contact with you. Please do not hesitate to contact me if you have further questions.

Summary

Attorneys are a vital and growing professional group in our culture. There is great potential for building mutual referral networks with them. Use the information and resources in this chapter to strategically begin building networks with the legal community. This information may also serve as a basis for research into the legal profession.

Resources

Internet

Access to an online computer can provide numerous resources. Most sites are user friendly and responsive. The following sites are a beginning for your Internet directory. Many of these sites have links to other sites of common professional interest. You may also use your Internet search tools for your particular areas of interest.

Bar Association and Other Web Sites

American Bar Association—www.abanet.org

Commission on Lawyer Assistance Programs—www.abanet.org/cpr/colap/home.html

Directory of Lawyer Assistance Programs—www.banet.org/cpr/colap/assistance.html

(You may download a national directory of LAP programs from their web site or send $25.00 to ABA Membership Services, 541 North Fairbanks Court, Chicago, IL, 60611; (312) 988-5359)

Divorce Online—www.divorceonline.com

Forensic Psychology—www.forensic-psych.com

Lawyer's Weekly (a highly informative national newspaper)—www.lawyersweekly.com/masslaw.html

National Lawyers Guild—www.nlg.org

States with Web Sites

Alabama State Bar Association—www.alabar.org

Alaska State Bar Association—www.alaskabar.org

Arizona State Bar Association—www.azbar.org

Arkansas Bar Association—www.arkbar.com

State Bar of California—www.calbar.org

Colorado Bar Association—www.cobar.org

Connecticut Bar Association—www.ctbar.org

Delaware State Bar Association—www.dsba.org
District of Columbia Bar Association—www.dcbar.org
Bar Association of District of Columbia—www.badc.org
The Florida Bar—www.flabar.org
State Bar of Georgia—www.gabar.org
Hawaii State Bar Association—www.hsba.org
Idaho State Bar Association—www2.stateid.us/isb
Illinois State Bar Association—www.illinoisbar.org
Iowa State Bar Association—www.iowabar.org/maininsf
Indiana State Bar—www.ai.org/isba
Kansas Bar Association—www.ksbar.org
Kentucky Bar Association—www.kybar.org
Louisiana State Bar—www.lsba.org
Maine State Bar—www.mainebar.org
Maryland State Bar Association—www.msba.org
Massachusetts Bar Association—www.massbar.org
State Bar of Michigan—www.michbar.org
Minnesota State Bar Association—www.mnbar.org
The Mississippi Bar—www.msbar.org
The Missouri Bar—www.mobar.org
Montana State Bar Association—www.montanabar.org
Nebraska State Bar Association—www.nebar.com
Nevada State Bar—www.nvbar.org
New Hampshire Bar Association—www.nhbar.org
New Jersey State Bar Association—www.njsba.com
New York State Bar—www.nysba.org
North Carolina Bar Association—www.barlinc.org
Ohio State Bar Association—www.ohio.bar.org
Oregon State Bar—www.osbar.org
Pennsylvania Bar Association—www.pabar.org
Rhode Island State Bar—www.ribar.com
State Bar of South Carolina—www.scbar.org
State Bar of South Dakota—www.sdbar.org
Tennessee Bar Association—www.tba.org/index.html

Texas State Bar Association—www.texasbar.com/start.htm

Utah State Bar—www.utahbar.org

Vermont Bar Association—www.vtbar.org

Virginia State Bar—www.vsb.org

Washington State Bar Association—www.wsba.org

West Virginia State Bar—www.wvbar.org

Wisconsin Bar Association—www.wisbar.org

Groups

American Bar Association
750 North Lake Shore Drive
Chicago, IL 60611
(312) 988-5000
Fax: (312) 988-5280

International Lawyers in Alcoholics Anonymous (ILAA)
200 South Third
Las Vegas, NV 89155
(702) 455-4711
Fax: (702) 383-8465

Legal Therapy Institute, Inc.
915 Gulf Tower, 707 Grant Street,
Pittsburgh, PA 15219
(412) 263-5636

National Academy of Elder Law Attorneys, Inc.
1604 North Country Club Lane
Tucson, AZ 85716
(520) 881-4005
Fax: (520) 325-7925

Publications

Lawyer's Weekly USA, 41 West Street, Boston, MA 02111 (800) 444-LAWS. Also available on the Internet—www.lawyersweekly.com/masslaw.html

Martindale-Hubbell International Law Directory (see Recommended Reading). Also available on the Internet—www.martindale.com

Black's Legal Dictionary (see Recommended Reading).

Recommended Reading

Becker, L.C. (Ed.). (1992). *Encyclopedia of ethics* (Vol. 1, pp. 653–663). New York and London: Garland.

Bell, S.J. (1989). *Full disclosure: Do you really want to be a lawyer?* Princeton, NJ: Peterson's Guides.

Benjamin, G.H., Kaszniak, A., Sales, B., & Shanfield, S.B. (1986). The role of legal education in producing psychological distress among law students and lawyers. *American Bar Foundation Research Journal, 2*, 225.

Black, H.C. (1933). *Black's law dictionary*. St. Paul, MN: West.

Bosoni, A.J. (1992). *Legal resource directory: A guide to free or inexpensive assistance for low income families, with special sections for prisoners;* Jefferson, NC and London: McFarland.

Daw, J. (Ed.). (1997–1998, December/January). *Divorce lawyers could use therapists. Family Therapy News*, 11, 27. Washington, DC: American Association for Marriage and Family Therapy.

Edwards, P. (Ed.). (1967). *The encyclopedia of philosophy* (Vol. 6, pp. 254–275). New York: Macmillan and Free Press.

Elwork, A. (1997). *Stress management for lawyers.* Gwynedd, PA: Vorkell Group.

Elwork, A., & Benjamin, G.A.H. (1995). Lawyers in distress. *Journal of Psychiatry and Law 23* (Summer), 205.

Encyclopedia Americana (International Ed.). (1972). (Vol. 17, pp. 71–79, 164–166). Danbury, CT: Grolier.

Foonberg, J.G. (1995). *Finding the right lawyer.* Chicago: American Bar Association.

Gifis, S.H. (1993). *Dictionary of legal terms: A simplified guide to the language of law* (2nd ed.). Hauppauge, NY: Barron's Educational Series.

Goetz, P.W. (Ed.). (1987). *The new encyclopaedia Britannica* (Vol. 7, pp. 200–201). Chicago: Encyclopaedia Britannica.

Goldberg, S.B. (1990). One in five lawyers dissatisfied. *American Bar Association Journal, 76*(10), 36.

Hastings, J. (Ed.). (1922). *Encyclopaedia of religion and ethics* (Vol. 7, p. 805–889). New York: Scribner's.

Hill, G.N., & Hill, K.T. (1995). *Real life dictionary of the law: Taking the mystery out of legal language.* Santa Monica, CA: General Publishing Group.

Kramer, S.N., & Eds. (1967). *Cradle of civilization.* New York: Time-Life Books.

Lawless, L.L. (1997). *Therapy, Inc.: A hands-on guide to developing, positioning, and marketing your practice in the 90s.* New York: Wiley.

Margulies, S. (1997). Representing the client from hell: Divorce and the borderline client. *Journal of Law and Psychiatry, 25*, 348.

Martindale-Hubbell American Arbitration Association. (1994). *Martindale-Hubbell dispute resolution directory.* New Providence, NJ: Author.

Martindale-Hubbell American Arbitration Association. (1995). *Martindale-Hubbell International Law Directory.* New Providence, NJ: Author.

McCormack, M.H. (1987). *The terrible truth about lawyers: How lawyers really work and how to deal with them successfully.* New York: Beech Tree Books, Morrow.

Moss, D.C. (1991). Lawyer personality. ABA *Journal 77*(2), 34.

Ostberg, K. (1985). *Using a lawyer . . . And what to do if things go wrong: A step by-step guide.* New York: Random House.

Richard, L.R. (1993). The lawyer types. ABA *Journal 79*(7), 74.

5

Strategies for Getting Referrals from Religious Leaders

Building referral systems with religious leaders has great potential for your practice. Statistics from the U.S. Department of Labor, published in 1992, indicate that there are approximately 312,000 clergy serving congregations (255,000 Protestant pastors, 4,000 rabbis, and 53,000 Roman Catholic priests). Not included in this number are clergy from other faiths and approximately 100,000 Roman Catholic nuns.

Clergy are often the first persons men and women turn to for help with problems.

Clergy are often the first contact for people who need help with problems. Although less than 10 percent of the men and women seeking counsel eventually receive referrals, most clergy make some referrals to mental health professionals. Clergy prefer to refer congregants or others who come for assistance to a therapist they know and trust. One study indicated that when clergy attend a workshop or seminar about mental health, their referral rates shoot up dramatically (Weaver, Koenig, & Larson, 1997).

Many people use their spirituality and religion as a major coping strategy to deal with life's traumas and transitions. The United States has approximately 500,000 houses of worship of all faiths. Gallup surveys (1990–1994) exploring religious patterns of Americans indicate that 40 percent of the population attend a house of worship on a weekly basis. In addition, 60 percent attend a house of worship at least once a month. About 90 percent occasionally pray (Weaver, Koenig, & Larson, 1997). As therapists, it is important to keep these statistics in mind as you consider the well-being of your clients and explore whether religion or spirituality is a positive or negative experience in their lives. Even if you choose not to build a referral network with the religious community, opening lines of communication to religious leaders can be helpful to you in working with clients who raise religious issues about which you are uninformed.

Religion is and continues to be a powerful force in individual lives and the American culture.

Religion is and continues to be a powerful force in individual lives. In our modern society, we have moved from a worldview in which religion was at the center to a worldview with the natural sciences at the center. Splits and controversies have occurred between the religious arena and the competing sciences, creating barriers between some religious leaders and mental health professionals. The range spans from open dialogue, to slight suspicion and mistrust, to downright antagonism. Mental health professionals who want to build networks with the religious community must understand and overcome these barriers.

Sigmund Freud, trained in the scientific worldview, is often understood by the religious community as a primary disrespector of religious faith due to his paradigm of religion as a residue of psychic development. Freud (1961) wrote:

> Our knowledge of the historical worth of certain religious doctrines increases our respect for them, but does not invalidate our proposal that they should cease to be put forward as the reasons for the precepts of civilization. On the contrary! Those historical residues have helped us to view religious teachings, as it were, as neurotic relics, and we may now argue that the time has probably come, as it does in an analytic treatment, for replacing the effects of repression by the results of the rational operation of the intellect. (p. 44)

This viewpoint has provoked tensions that make networking with religious leaders problematic. Being prepared to respond to such issues will increase the likelihood of receiving referrals from the religious community. A helpful book that explores these issues and includes essays from acknowledged authorities in the field is *Religion and the Clinical Practice of Psychology* (Shafranske, 1996).

Characteristics of the Clergy

To build ongoing relationships with religious leaders, you need to understand who they are.

To build ongoing relationships with religious leaders, you need to understand who they are. Although there is no one profile for clergy, there are characteristics important to successful ministry. The great majority of clergy have a bachelor's degree and a master of divinity degree. The master of divinity is a three-year post-bachelor's degree. Statistics from Andover Newton Theological School (MA), the oldest theological school in the United States show that a recent student body totaling 477 was composed of 60 percent women and 40 percent men. The student body was composed of 12 percent ethnic minorities and/or international students. The majority of their seminarians were second-career students and the average age was 40. Many clergy have postgraduate degrees, such as a Doctor of Ministry (DMin), a PhD, or a Master of Sacred Theology (STM). Contact seminaries, theological schools, or denominational offices in your region to gain a composite picture of religious leaders in your vicinity and their requirements for ordination. Or have a conversation with a local clergy about what is required for ordination to professional religious leadership.

Cox (1985) maintains that most successful religious leaders maintain a solid sense of identity, have the ability to form true friendships, are highly empathic, and can tolerate ambiguity. Clergy are also receptive to continuing education opportunities that enhance their pastoral abilities although they are not required to have a certain number of CEUs to maintain ordination status.

As with many other professionals, stress levels are high for those in professional religious leadership. In a study conducted by the United Church of Christ as to why men leave parish ministry, clergy gave the following reasons (in order of primacy):

> . . . a sense of personal and professional inadequacy, . . . unable to relocate when necessary, problems of wife and children, lack of opportunity to put training and skill to fullest use, personal illness or breakdown, dissatisfaction with parish work, lack of church's spiritual growth and relevance was stultifying, divorce or separation, money problems, more attractive job opportunity, and other reasons. (Cox, 1985)

These issues, including those involved in success as well as those involved in career dissatisfactions, provide opportunities and potential to the mental health professional for developing services and products focused on professional religious leaders.

Because both the clergy and the mental health professional desire to promote the well-being of others, there is much common ground in their work. Demythologizing the professions can be helpful to all of us. As you relate to clergy, name the attributes you share with them in helping people with problems. This will assist communication and the building of common ground.

Demythologizing the professions can be helpful to all of us.

The Marketplace

You will find it easy to locate and contact most clergy. The majority of congregations have less than 100 members, and many do not have on-site full-time clerical assistance. The Alban Institute tested 1,319 clergy of various denominations regarding their Myers-Briggs Personality Type and found that 61 percent were extroverted (Oswald & Kroeger, 1988). This means the majority of clergy enjoy engaging with others. Your initial communication to them, whether by letter or by telephone, has a high probability of evoking a response. If not, follow up with a telephone call. At the same time, remember that clergy have busy schedules; respect their time constraints.

Many clergy and denominations are confronted by declining congregational membership and a spiritually competitive field that includes immigrant and ethnic communities, Eastern and esoteric religious groups, and community groups vying for volunteers. Competition for pastoral positions also is intense, salaries are low, and many graduates have accumulated high educational debt. Congregations are closing their doors and selling properties. Downsizing and mergers are occurring, and congregations are hiring part-time or bivocational clergy because they often cannot afford a full-time pastor. These factors add great stress to the life of the religious professional. These crises provide opportunities for mental health professionals to be understanding and empathic toward clergy as well as to develop services for them.

Ordained clergy and other professional religious leaders also serve in specialized ministries (nonparish settings). Examples of nonparish settings are hospital, military, prison, and college chaplaincies; social ministries (neighborhood centers, housing and feeding services, etc.); mission work; denominational administration; higher education; and pastoral counseling centers.

Clergy are often involved with men, women, families, and communities at their most celebrative moments as well as at their most vulnerable.

Market Future

Clergy are often involved with men, women, families, and communities at their most celebrative moments—weddings, births, baptisms, installations of leaders—as well as at their most vulnerable—illness, death, loss, posttrauma, divorce, community and national calamities. They support and help people as they maneuver life's transitions. It can be difficult for clergy to provide long-term, consistent pastoral care to congregants (particularly if the clergy is part-time or bivocational); therefore, clergy may be receptive to making referrals to mental health professionals that they know in the community. Since these events are continuous and ongoing in life, the future is bright for collaboration between clergy and mental health professionals.

Market Needs

In a 1986 study of 2,000 Protestant pastors, 95 percent of whom had received some counseling education in seminary, only 39 percent felt competent in areas of mental health and family counseling (Orthner, 1986). Clergy indicated the need for skill building in the areas of referral and diagnostic skills as well as a greater understanding of mental health issues for the elderly and their family dynamics. They expressed a need for additional training in the following areas (Weaver, Koenig & Larsen, January 1997): ". . . . marriage and family problems, divorce and separation, parenting problems, marital counseling, child or spouse abuse, counseling singles, sexual adjustment, remarriage/step family, and premarital counseling and the elderly."

Mental health professionals can provide services and products in these areas. Community organizations seeking speakers or workshop facilitators also often use pastors as a resource. Networking with the religious community may well provide possible referrals.

Competition

Pastoral counselors are an interfaith group with which you may choose to network. Pastoral counselors are clergy, rabbis, or religious (of the Roman Catholic tradition) who have Master of Divinity degrees and have also obtained a degree in psychiatry, psychology, counseling, social work, or pastoral counseling.

The major accrediting body for pastoral counselors is the American Association of Pastoral Counselors

The major accrediting body for pastoral counselors is the American Association of Pastoral Counselors (AAPC), an interfaith organization. Many clergy are also members of the American Association of Marriage and Family Therapists (AAMFT). Another group composed of clergy and mental health professionals is the American Association of Christian Counselors (AACC; see Resources).

Look in the Yellow Pages to see whether there are listings for Pastoral Counselors or Christian Counselors; check with the previously listed organizations for member listings in your area and also ask pastors if there are pastoral counselors in the area to whom they now refer congregants. Add these names to your contact list and mail your Resource Directory Worksheet to them, along with your brochure, business card, and mail-back card. This is a way to begin networking with these like-minded mental health professionals.

Your Experiences with the Clergy

Your educational experiences and the attitudes of your professors and professional models will also influence your beliefs about religious communities.

Almost everyone has a history with a religious community and its leaders. These experiences—good, bad, indifferent, ugly—have created your intellectual and emotional stance toward them. It is important to remember your family's experience with religious personages and organizations as well. As a mental health professional, your educational experiences and the attitudes of your professors and professional models will also influence your beliefs about religious communities. When you have completed the following section, ask yourself if you can honestly work with professional religious leaders while maintaining your sense of integrity.

To be successful in building referral networks with clergy, first try to find those with whom you share areas of like-mindedness. To do this, you need to review your own background.

Making a Match

Refer to your family-of-origin genogram to focus on you and your family-of-origin's religious history to answer the questions in the following seven areas:

1. Were you baptized, christened, or dedicated as a baby or young child? Do you have a certificate indicating such a ritual took place? Where is the certificate? Did you have a bar mitzvah or bat mitzvah? Were you circumcised? Were you confirmed? Are there photographs/films/videos of any of the above? Who has and where are the records?

2. Did you attend religious services; are you a member of a religious congregation? What type? How long? With whom did/do you attend? Did you participate in religious education classes? What do you remember about them? How did the instructor respond to your questions? Did you like attending or were you made to go? Favorite teachers?
3. What are/were your feelings about the pastor/priest/sister/rabbi? Are any family members professional religious leaders?
4. Did you and/or your siblings attend religious based schools? Feelings about that?
5. What were/are your parents' beliefs? What is their religion? What religious practices did you observe at home and in the community? Did their parents (your grandparents) involve them in any activities listed in questions 1 and 2? What were/are parental attitudes to religious practices? How does/did the family manage marriages and funerals? Decisions about career? What were/are family responses to historical events such as natural disasters, war, and other catastrophes?
6. Out of the mosaic of you and your family's religious traditions, what beliefs and traditions do you perceive about yourself and divinity in the midst of your daily existence?
7. If your family did not practice any religious tradition, how did you feel about that? What are your current thoughts/feelings/practices regarding the religious or spiritual life?

Having insight and understanding into your personal dynamics and experiences as they relate to religion and/or spirituality will be helpful in networking and communicating with religious leaders. See if you can place yourself somewhere on the bell curve shown in Figure 5.1. Doing so can help you decide where and how you might begin entering into relationships with those in religious communities. This will assist in locating those with whom you may be more like-minded.

Locating Yourself on the Religious Expressions Diagram

Figure 5.1 develops a range of religious expressions. Most of you will probably fall somewhere within the middle of the curve. If so, you will

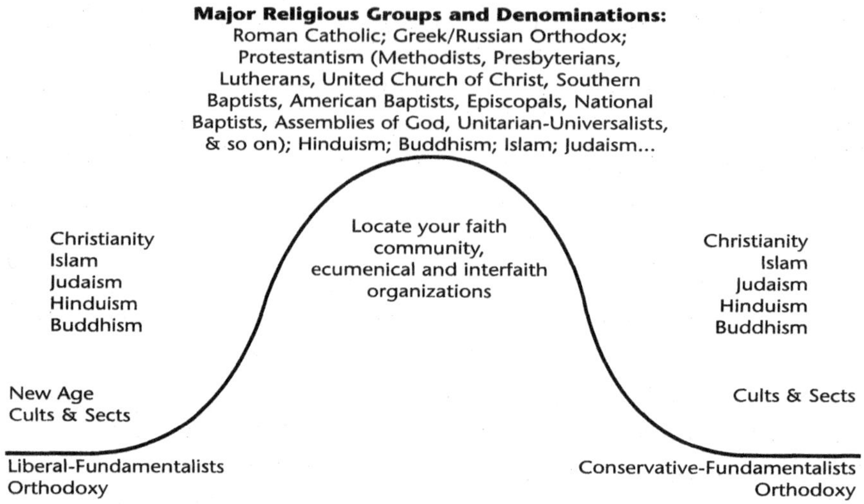

FIGURE 5.1 Religious Bell Curve

want to contact clergy who are serving congregations in the middle or the more liberal traditions. If you are on either end of the curve, you may want to review belief systems of the other groupings before contacting them (see Resources for suggestions).

Being comfortable with your own spirituality, your religious history, and your therapeutic family identities will communicate a positive sense of who you are and the philosophy with which you approach your clients.

Your Therapeutic "Family"

Review Figure 1.2. Refamiliarize yourself with the schools of thought with which you are most related and committed. Are you most comfortable with the existentialist thinking of the Rollo May school? Carl Jung and the Jungians? Family systems thinking? Cognitive Behavioral? Rogerian? Relational psychology? Locate yourself among the various schools and practice telling the story of your "therapy family" roots. Clergy will want to know this, and the more you are able to share such information, the more trust and confidence you will build with them. Being comfortable with your own spirituality, your religious history, and your therapeutic family identities will communicate a positive sense of who you are and the philosophy with which you approach your clients.

Engaging the Marketplace

Creating a Mindmap

After you have completed the preceding section and feel confident that you want to develop networks with the religious community, use the sample mindmap illustrated in Figure 5.2 as a guide for developing your own map for researching the information you will need. Be attentive to the sensibilities and particularities of your community and region.

Creating a Goal-Setting Worksheet

A goal-setting worksheet (refer to Figure 2.4) will lead you in choosing what you want to do and when you plan to do it. It provides self-accountability for you in beginning and developing your bridges to the religious community.

Niche Areas

If you have expertise in any marketable niche areas, develop your materials along those lines. Religious communities often have adult education opportunities and are often looking for speakers; don't hesitate to offer your expertise in these services.

Services and Products

As you build relationships with the religious community, listen carefully and take the initiative in offering your talents and skills. When you make presentations or facilitate workshops, remember to have brochures and flyers with you for distribution to those in attendance.

You can divide potential services and products into at least three categories: (1) offerings for clergy; (2) offerings for the congregation as a whole, such as workshops, seminars, retreats; (3) offerings for individual congregational members, couples, and families. The latter services/products will be focused on your therapeutic specialties. Consider the possibilities for development in each category using the following suggestions to fuel your creativity.

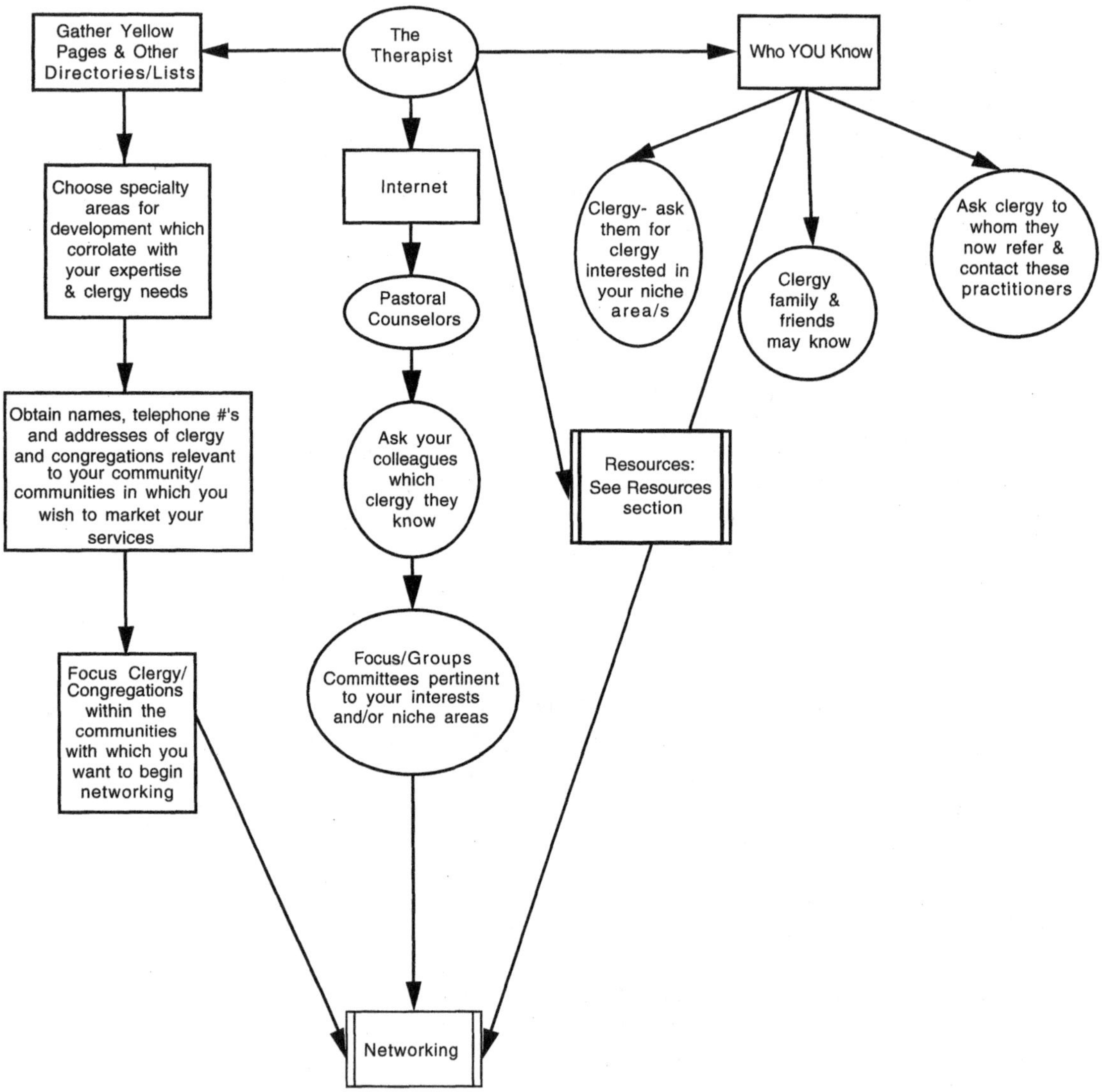

FIGURE 5.2 Mindmap for Developing a Network in Religious Communities

Offerings to Clergy

- *Continuing Education and/or Workshop Events.* Most clergy do not need to have continuing education units to maintain their professional status. They are, however, very interested in increasing their skills.

- *Presentations/Speaker.* Clergy are often looking for speakers for special congregational services and programs that occur around the religious seasons such as:
  - Ecumenical or interfaith Thanksgiving services.
  - Advent season (the four Sundays prior to Christmas); for example, workshop/presentation addressing holiday stresses, the "blues," the meaning of gifts and money.
  - Lenten season (the six weeks prior to Easter; many congregations sponsor a weekly series of events with selected speakers and topics); for example, a workshop focusing on topics such as betrayal, reconciliation, forgiveness, suffering, grief and loss, managing of pain, meditation and healing, possibilities for emotional and spiritual growth via life challenges.
  - Children's Sundays (often in June).
  - Mother's Day and Father's Day (May and June).
  - Mental Health Month (May; see Resources).
  - Mental Health Awareness Week (October; see Resources).
  - Friday evening programs at Reformed and Conservative synagogues to which they may invite speakers.
- *Peer Supervision.* Facilitate small groups for clergy case presentation.
- *Written Materials.* Offer an article for the congregational newsletter, or offer an "Ask the Counselor" column. Or allow copying of the feature article in your newsletter with acknowledgment of its source including your name, address, and telephone number.

Offerings to the Entire Congregation and/or Groups

Developing and offering presentations to congregational groups can be another powerful way of building a client base, and the clergy is most often the gatekeeper to these opportunities. Some examples for different congregational groups are:

Women's Groups

Overcoming Depression
Phases of Life Transitions
Thriving in Midlife

Men's Groups

Stages of a Man's Life
Stress Reduction
Male Generativity

Couples Groups

Venus and Mars, Is It So?
Two-Career Families
The Sandwich Generation

Parent Groups

Building Self-Esteem in Children and Adolescents
Raising a Moral Child
Communication Skills and Discipline
Building Romance into Relationships

Youth Groups—Junior and Senior High Youth

Negotiating with Adults
Building Trust with Others
Dating Relationships
Say "No" and Keep Your Friends
How to Be a Friend

Young Adult Groups

Dating Relationships
Couple Development
How to Fight Fair
Two-Career Relationships
Positive Ways to Deal with Loneliness

Play Groups

Building Esteem in Your Child
Self-Care of Mom
Parenting Resources in the Community

Community Groups

Alcoholics Anonymous
Overeaters Anonymous
Singles
Parents without Partners
(12-Step groups often use church space for their meetings. They may approach the pastor about potential speakers.)

Congregational Boards and Committees

Leadership Skill Building
Communication Tools for Effective Meetings
Myers-Briggs Type Indicator and Team-Building

Offerings to Individual Members of the Congregation and Other Related Groups

When you are invited to make presentations or to lead an adult education event or workshop to a group, board, or committee, always have your brochures available along with flyers about any groups or programs you are offering. Arrange the brochures on a table at the meeting location for those who are interested and point out their availability. These outreach materials will describe your therapeutic specialties (e.g., marriage and family, child/adolescent, group therapy, blended families, sex educator). The pastor will most often be a gatekeeper for members of the congregation so distribute brochures and cards to the clergy. Following your presentation, be available to attendees who may have questions and also distribute your outreach materials to them. This is a natural location to begin building trusting relationships with persons who may want to use your services at some future time or who may refer their friends and family members to you.

The pastor will most often be a gatekeeper for members of the congregation so distribute brochures and cards to the clergy.

Additionally, the person who will be opening the presentation may ask how to introduce you. Have a written piece available for this purpose. In the introductory material, state your specialty areas and services/products for individuals, couples, and families. If no one asks you for introductory material, offer the information and share that you have biographical material they may want to use in making the introduction. Repetition reinforces memory, and you want your services and products to be remembered.

Outreach Vehicles

As you develop and create your outreach vehicles, you may use the following as models for your own creativity. Consider your location, its economic status, and the religious communities that will read your materials. Place yourself in the position of the reader or respondent to your services and products, and ask yourself if the material would attract or invite your response. Is it speaking to the needs of the reader? Often, when mental health professionals develop their materials, they unknowingly direct them toward their peers rather than the potential consumers of the services. In the case of these outreach materials, the potential client will be someone within a faith community. Develop your marketing materials accordingly. Know as much about the local faith communities as possible prior to developing outreach materials.

Develop your marketing materials accordingly. Know as much about the local faith communities as possible prior to developing outreach materials.

If you have a computer and a desktop publishing program, it is easy to develop and print your brochures and most of the following outreach vehicles. This also reduces expenses. If you do not as yet have the necessary computer technology, then a local printing company will be able to do this for you at a fairly reasonable rate. Limit your printings so that you may adapt and/or update them on a regular basis. When you do a new client intake, always ask how the person or group learned about you and your services. This information will help you identify which outreach vehicles are most productive. You will want to create the following practice outreach resources:

- *Brochure.* Acknowledge on the brochure that you are specifically responding to those who value faith as an important element of their lifestyle. Clearly state your respect for such values. Use your general brochure for distribution to congregational members and to clergy, along with business cards. Give a supply to the clergy for use with those whom they might want to refer. Figure 5.3 shows a sample brochure.
- *Cover Letter and Other Types of Letters.* Letters, along with the other outreach vehicles, maintain a visible presence for your products and services. They also aid name recognition. Consistent presence adds tremendously to your practice development and viability as a mental health professional. Your products/services are needed. Be proactive in offering them. Figures 5.4 and 5.5 show sample letters.
- *Resource Directory Worksheet for Clergy.* Although you may decide not to actively seek networking with clergy, having the clergy resource information on hand may be an important adjunct to supporting clients with spiritual questions or issues. It is wise to update this information on a yearly basis. The average length of a pastorate is 5 to 7 years, and you will want to remain current with the available pastoral resources. Figure 5.6 shows a useful format for a worksheet.
- *Newsletter.* When you mail your newsletter to the local clergy, request a copy of one of their church newsletters. You may also request a copy of their state/national denominational newsletter. Request to be added to the mailing list. Such information will keep you informed as to relevant issues in the local, state, and national faith communities. (It is courteous to make a contribution toward mailing costs.) Give permission for them to use any of your newsletter items in their newsletter; ask that they identify the source of the information.
- *Business Card.* Direct the business card content to the specific professional group with whom you wish to network. Just as with the

The Alpha Centre offers Clergy and their congregational members assistance with counseling and/or locating needed resources. We ar sensitive to and respectful of religious values.

Call 781.322.3051 for

Individual Counseling and Personal Growth
By considering interpersonal behaviors in your relationships and work experiences, and gaining awareness of your relational style and goals, new options and resources may be developed.

Family Therapy
By exploring relationship patterns, the family may develop healthier styles of relating and dealing with problems.

Workshop and Retreat Leadership
We will team with you in planning and facilitating a program and process which will be forward you goals for a successful group experience.

Couples Counseling
Couples are assisted in clarifying their hopes and expectations of the relationship, enhancing communication skills, and co-creating the type of relationship they desire.

Separation Counseling and/or Divorce Mediation
When a relationship must end, impartial caring mediation can help you take charge of arrangements, avoid unnecessary injury to spouses and children, and save an average of 90% of the cost of litigated divorce.

Professional Consultation
If you are wondering what to do about a situation and would like an objective viewpoint and/or resources or referrals, we will work with you in reaching your goals.

The Alpha Centre

Sliding Fee Scale available for Uninsured and Private Pay Clients

---

Accessible by Public Transportation (Take the Bus or The Orange Line to Malden Center)

Parking Available On-street and in Parking Garages or Parking Lots

---

Elevator Building
Handicap Accessible

Directions by car to Malden:

Rt. 60 East to Main Street; turn left onto Main Street and take the second left onto Pleasant Street; 6 Pleasant Street is at the corner of Main and Pleasant Street

The Alpha Centre
6 Pleasant St. Ste. 214
Malden MA 02148

Phone: 781.322.5051
Fax: 781.662.8575

It is a sign of wisdom, not weakness, to ask for help.

The Alpha Centre

the resource for you when you're seeking support with the programming and pastoral needs of your congregation, and are looking for attitudes sensitvie to, and respectful of religious values

The Alpha Centre

Linda L Lawless, MA

Licensed

Marriage Family Therapist

Mental Health counselor

Certified Group Psychotherapist

You will find my counseling approach thoughtful and supportive. I combine clinical training and 20 years of counseling experience with real caring to ease you through the "bumpy spots" of life. Current specialities include: low self-esteem, life transitions (menopause, career change, divorce); recovery from trauma (physical and/or psychological abuse, incest); food and weight problems; and stress management. Women's groups available. M.A. (Clinical Psychology) from J.F. Kennedy University, Orinda CA. Co-Founder, Alpha Centre. Author of *Therapy, Inc* 1997 Wiley & Sons NY.

The Alpha Centre

Jean Wright, D.Min.

Licensed

Marriage and Family Therapist

Mental Health Counselor

American Baptist Clergy

My specialities include counseling with those who suffer from the aftereffects of abuse and trauma, and those who are experiencing panic, depression, anxiety, or stressful changes in their lives. I also assist couples and families around communication, decision-making, and step-family issues. Another focus area is that of job and career and helping men and women find that which is meaningful to their life. I also work with people who have spiritual or religious concerns. A trained family and divorce mediator, I assist couples to manage the processes involved in separation and divorce in a non-adversarial manner. D. Min. from Andover Newton Theological School. Co-Founder of Alpha Centre. Unpublished D.Min. paper: "And God Laughed: Pastoral Counseling and Therapeutic Humor."

Linda and Jean are available for speaking engagements, workshops, seminars and retreat facilitation

When you're looking for program resources to support your ministry

The Alpha Centre works with Institutions and Businesses in developing educational training programs. We offer workshops, seminars, and presentations in the areas listed below. We work with you in customizing programs to meet your needs.

Stress Management

Communication Skills

Team-Building

Conflict Mediation & Resolution

Goal Setting & Strategic Planning

Improving Motivation and Morale

Problem-Solving

Wholistic Well-Being

Laughter Training

Raising a Moral Child

Building Self-Esteem In Children

Call 781-322-3051 to arrange an informational meeting

The Alpha Centre Mission Statement

Our mission is to be a professional resource in support of the health and well-being of

- the whole person
- families
- business, institutions, and municipalities

in the service of creating caring community

When you or someone whom you care about is hurting in areas of

The Alpha Centre offers clergy and their congregational members assistance with counseling and/or locating needed resources. We are sensitive to and respectful of religious values.

- Addiction
- Sexual issues
- Financial stress
- Work-related problems
- Memories of abuse
- Unresolved bereavement
- Separation and divorce
- Lack of friends, troubled relationships
- Aging, and/or chronic physical or emotional illness
- Personal inner hurt, fear, sadness, depression, or anger
- Parenting, step-parenting, and family relationships

The Alpha Centre
6 Pleasant St. Ste. 214
Malden Ma 02148
781.322.3051

FIGURE 5.3 Example Brochure for Congregational Members and Clergy

Alpha Centre

6 Pleasant Street Suite 214 Malden MA 02148 617-322-3051

Our mission is to be a professional resource in support of the health and well-being of
- *The whole person*
- *Families*
- *Businesses, institutions, and*
- *Municipalities*

in the service of creating caring community

BUILDING SELF-ESTEEM IN CHILDREN

RAISING A MORAL CHILD

COMMUNICATION SKILLS AND CONFLICT MANAGEMENT

STAGES OF FAITH DEVELOPMENT

HUMOR IN THE BIBLE

SKILLS FOR STRESS MANAGEMENT AND REDUCTION

HOW TO MAKE REFERRALS

BEING A SUCCESSFUL SINGLE

SURVIVING AND THRIVING AS A STEP-FAMILY

CENTERING PRAYER: LISTENING TO GOD

MENTAL ILLNESS: WHAT IS IT?

AGING AS A SPIRITUAL JOURNEY

HOW TO CHOOSE THE RIGHT THERAPIST

CREATING LIFESTYLE CHANGE

Dear __________:

I am currently seeing a parishioner of yours, Frank Smith. He entered counseling to deal with issues regarding his recent divorce. The attached release allows us to discuss his case freely.

Mr. Smith is having some difficulty integrating his faith with the reality of his divorce. I've suggested that he be in touch with you to discuss these faith concerns and have shared with him that I would be contacting you.

I believe it will be helpful to Mr. Smith to have your pastoral support at this time. Please do not hesitate to contact me if you have any questions, and I will be in touch with you by telephone regarding Mr. Smith's progress.

Sincerely,

FIGURE 5.4 Sample Letter to Clergy about Seeing a Parishioner

Dear __________:

On September 17, 1999, I will be starting a monthly group (September-May) for clergy who would like to be part of an on-going case presentation seminar and wish to bring this to your attention should you want to participate. I am a licensed marriage and family therapist, with over twelve years experience and will facilitate the group.

The group will be limited to 8 clergy and will meet for 90 minutes the last Friday of each month, 1:30 - 3:00 PM. Cost per session will be ten dollars.

Format of the group will be as follows:

1. Opening - catch-up with group members; any business of the group.
   30 minutes
2. Case Presentations and Discussion. (Presentation dates will be voluntarily chosen).
   I will present a case at the first session.
3. Wrap-up and Adjournment.

The group members will serve as peer supervisors. Meeting discussions will be confidential.

Enclosed is an announcement, brochure, and newsletter.

If you wish to sign-up or have any questions, please contact me at (781) 322-3051.

Sincerely,

FIGURE 5.5 Sample Letter Announcing the Start-Up of a Group

Date: ________________ New: ________ Revision: ________

Name: ____

Congregation: ____

If Pastoral Counselor, Name of Practice: ________________________

Office Hours: ________________________________

Type of Practice: ________________________________

Specialties: ________________________________

Fees: Indicate if you use a sliding fee scale or other forms of payment options (e.g., credit cards, payment plans): ________________

Address: ____

Telephone(s): ____

Fax: ________________________ E-mail Address: ____________________

Web site: ____

Year Graduated Seminary: ________________ School: ____________________

Professional Memberships: ____

____

Languages Spoken: ____

Wheel Chair Accessible: Yes: ________ No: ________

What else is important for us to know about you or your congregation/training?

____

Thank you for completing this Resource Directory Form:

Please mail to:

Alpha Centre, 6 Pleasant Street, Suite 214, Malden, MA 02148. If you have any questions, please call (781-322-3051)

Linda Lawless, MA LMFT/LMHC/CCT; Jean Wright, D.Min, LMFT/LMHC

Source: Adapted from L. Lawless *Therapy Inc.* (New York: John Wiley, 1997). Reprinted with permission.

FIGURE 5.6 Clergy and/or Pastoral Counselor Resource Directory Worksheet

Telephone Script

Preparing. The clergyperson you are calling has received your letter and brochure in advance:

- Have the letter and brochure before you.
- Review your family-of-origin genogram and your bell curve of religious groupings as well as the way you will present your therapeutic style.
- Review the religion section of your local and area newspaper.
- Call when you are feeling refreshed.
- Take a deep breath and place the call. One of the following three possibilities will unfold.

Connecting:

1. You reach the answering machine. If so, identify yourself and confirm that you will call again. You may also request that the clergyperson telephone you (leave your telephone number) and if you aren't available to state times when he or she will be in the office. Do not hesitate to call again. Remember that most clergy are friendly but busy professionals. Also, remember that repetition aids retention.
2. You reach the church secretary (most of whom are quite helpful) and the cleric is not available: Identify yourself and request that the cleric return your call and/or leave times when you will be available. Calendar in a date to call again if there is no response.
3. You reach the clergyperson. Have your script at hand and follow it. Keep your text to one page and remember that the call is about building a relationship. Adapt the script to the particular call (i.e., this may be a cleric who returned the mail-back card showing interest in your programs and offerings). In your first paragraph, you begin building the relationship. Introduce yourself and your business and mention that you are a credentialed mental health professional:

> This is ______ of ______. I'm a licensed ______ and have been located in ______ since ______. How long have you been serving at ______? [You may want to make mention of information you have regarding the congregation or religious leader.]

Presentation. This makes up the second paragraph and contains your reason for calling:

> Did you receive the letter and brochure I mailed on ______? Do you have questions, comments about it?

The clergy may ask about your religious background and therapeutic style at this time and/or you may initiate it. Share why you want to network with clergy and that you believe you share a mutual desire to assist others. Mention common ground between the two professions (assisting and building a healthy community). You may also base comments on your mission statement. Invite the cleric's ideas about common ground.

(Continued)

- Ask if he or she is will assist you by sharing the mailing list of religious leaders in the community.
- Ask if there is a regular monthly ecumenical or interfaith meeting of the clergy and if you might be invited to that meeting. Can he or she be helpful or is there another contact? If so, who is that person?

Close. The third paragraph brings closure to the telephone meeting. Ask for an appointment to meet and further discuss how you might assist one another. Make appropriate thank-yous and close with a "looking forward to meeting you in person" statement. Follow up with a note.

Affirming. Give yourself a pat on the back! You're on your way to building a niche market.

Completing. Follow up the telephone call with a note stating that you appreciate the time taken and that you look forward to the possibility of working together around your common interests. If you have scheduled a luncheon meeting and/or appointment to meet, mention it.

brochure, identify yourself as a mental health professional respectful of and sensitive to faith values and concerns.

- *Mail-back Card.* Always remember that communication is interactive. Invite responses to your outreach and marketing materials.
- *Advertisement for Denominational or Congregational Newsletters.* Fees are often very affordable. If you place an advertisement in a local congregational newsletter, you may choose to rotate it among the various congregations over the course of a year. Your products/services will reach a larger audience and you will support the religious diversity inherent in most towns and cities.
- *Telephone Script.* Develop a telephone script (or use it face-to-face) such as the one shown on pages 147–148. It will help you explain your stance regarding religion to religious leaders as you meet and introduce yourself. It will be an important and helpful element in building bridges to the professional religious community.
- *"To Do" List.* The To Do checklist (see page 149) keeps you accountable with your goals. When you select the dates for

To Do List

- Gather Yellow Pages for your location and towns directly adjacent by [date].
- Look under religious organizations or churches and select the ones you will call first to make an appointment for meeting and to receive a directory of religious groups in your locale by [date].
- Ask to be invited to the next ecumenical or interfaith clergy meeting by [date].
- Offer to make a presentation about your work. These groups are often looking for presenters, usually for fairly informal luncheon or coffee gatherings by [date]. Take brochures, business cards, newsletters, and so on as handouts. Dress in a professional, businesslike manner.
- Send thank-you notes to the clergy who extended an invitation to the first meeting and copies of the directory/directories by [date].
- Prepare mailing to professional religious leaders by [date].
- Develop brochure by [date].
- Write cover letters by [date].
- Develop and write enclosures by [date].
- Develop and write newsletter by [date].
- Mail packet by [date].
- Schedule follow-up calls by [date].
- Practice sharing your religious story. Review genogram and religious bell curve.
- Practice sharing your therapeutic roots and practices (i.e., how you work and the why behind it).
- Develop questions to ask the clergy about their particular religious tradition. Examples: "What do you enjoy about your vocation?" "What issues do you find most concerning or interesting to your congregation?" "What are the basic beliefs of your tradition?"

completion, also note them in your personal calendar. Schedule the date and time for working on the components just as you would schedule a client. Do not overload. Be honest with yourself about your work style and your needs for assistance in completing your tasks. Get the help you need. Affirm yourself as each "to do" becomes "done."

Summary

It is important for therapists to understand faith and spirituality in considering the well-being of the whole person. It can be helpful to know whether religion or spirituality is a negative experience in the life of your client or whether it is a positive, life-enhancing attribute. It is useful to know if your clients pray or meditate. Building networks with clergy is a way not only to grow your practice but also to create avenues of communication that can enhance your therapeutic competency.

Being comfortable with your own spirituality, your religious history, and your therapeutic family identities will communicate a positive sense of who you are and how you became that person. Such self-presentation aids building relationships with clergy.

Although you don't need to be an expert, you do need to learn about the workings of congregations. Read about and talk with representatives of the various faith traditions (see Recommended Reading). Allow the faith communities to teach you about their ethos. Become a learner. Respect core values of the faith communities. Consider using a sliding fee structure if you do not already do so. Go for it. Be visible.

Resources

Professional Organizations

American Association of Christian Counselors (AACC)
P.O. Box 739
Forest, VA 24551
(800) 526-8673
Fax: (804) 384-3724
www.aacc.net

American Association of Pastoral Counselors (AAPC)
9504-A Lee Highway
Fairfax, VA 22031-2303
(703) 385-6967
Fax: (703) 352-7725
www.aapc.org

American Psychiatric Association (APA)
Committee on Religion and Psychiatry
1400 K Street, NW
Washington, DC 20077-1676
(202) 682-6000
www.psych.org

An excellent resource available from the APA and entitled *Mental Illnesses Awareness Guide for Clergy* has information for educating clergy and congregations. It is helpful for the preparation of presentations and workshops. Video resources are also listed.

Mental Health Awareness Week is in October.

May is Mental Health Awareness Month.

American Psychological Association
750 First Street, NE
Washington, DC 20002
(202) 336-5500
www.apa.org

Christian Association for Psychological Studies
P.O. Box 310400
New Braunfels, TX 78131-0400
(830) 629-2277
www.caps.net

The religion section of local and city newspapers often has a calendar of religious activities in the town and/or area and will offer additional information for use in talking with religious leaders.

For Consultation

Denice Adcock Colson, LPC, LMFT, CTRC
Trauma Education and Consultation Services
1603 Highway 16E
Jackson, Georgia 30233
(770) 504-8469

Denice works with clergy and congregations around trauma and abuse issues. She has authored a book *Victim to Victory: Resolving Past Trauma*, Trauma Education & Consultation Services, Pearland, TX, 1996, which she uses as a primary resource. Denice also consults to therapists.

Mark White, PhD
MFT Center, Glanton House
Auburn University
Auburn, AL 36849
(334) 844-4479
e-mail: mwhite@humsci.auburn.edu.

Mark is a professor in marriage and family therapy at Auburn University, Auburn, Alabama. He is of the Mormon tradition (The Church of Latter Day Saints—LDS) and a resource for those who work with that faith community.

Internet

The following have a wide range of information and links to denominational as well as other related sites such as Mind, Body, Spirit areas.

www.web.net/~ccchurch/other.html

www.ontario.anglican.ca/ecumenical.htm

www.ncccusa.org

www.ecunet.org/ecunet/ecuhome.htm

www.christiancounseling.org

Recommended Reading

Alexander, D., & Alexander, P. (Eds.). (1973). *Eerdmans' handbook to the Bible*. Grand Rapids, MI: Eerdmans.

Beaver, R.P., Bergman, J., Langey, M.S., Metz, W., Romarheim, A., Walls, A., Withycombe, R., & Wootton, R.W.F. (Eds.). (1982). *Eerdmans' handbook to the world's religions*. Grand Rapids, MI: Eerdmans.

Booth, L. (1991). *When God becomes a drug: Breaking the chains of religious addiction and abuse*. Los Angeles: Tarcher.

Brinton, C. (Ed.). (1969). *The portable age of reason reader*. New York: Viking Press.

Carver, T. (Ed.). (1997). *The Cambridge companion to Marx*. Cambridge, England: Cambridge University Press.

Cox, R.G. (1985). *Do you mean me, Lord? The call to the ordained ministry*. Philadelphia: Westminster Press.

Dowley, T. (Ed.). (1997). *Eerdmans' handbook to the history of Christianity*. Grand Rapids, MI: Eerdmans.

Droege, T.A. (1983). *Faith passages and patterns*. Philadelphia: Fortress Press.

Fowler, J., & Keen, S. (1978). *Life maps: Conversations on the journey of faith*. Waco, TX: Word Books.

Fowler, J., & Keen, S. (1981). *Stages of faith, the psychology of human development and the quest for meaning*. San Francisco: Harper & Row.

Freud, S. (1961). *The future of an illusion* (J. Strachey, Ed. & Trans.). New York: Norton.

Freud, S. (1961). *Civilization and its discontents* (J. Strachey, Ed. & Trans.). New York: Norton.

Fromm, E. (1978). *Psychoanalysis & religion*. New Haven, CT: Yale University Press.

Gleason, J.J., Jr. (1981). *Consciousness and the ultimate*. Nashville, TN: Abingdon.

Hirsch, E.D., Jr., Kett, J.F., & Trefil, J. (1988). *The dictionary of cultural literacy: What every American needs to know*. Boston: Houghton Mifflin.

Jung, C.G. (1966). *Psychology and religion*. New Haven, CT: Yale University Press.

Keirsey, D., & Bates, M. (1984). *Please understand me: Character and temperament types.* Del Mar, CA: Gnosology Books.

Lawless, L.L. (1997). Therapy, Inc. A hands-on guide to developing, practicing, and marketing your mental health practice in the 90s.

Levinson, J.C. (1993). *Guerrilla marketing: Secrets for making big profits from your small business.* New York and Boston: Houghton Mifflin.

Marx, K., & Engels, F. (1985). *The Communist manifesto.* London: Penguin Books.

McGoldrick, M., & Gerson, R. (1985). *Genograms in family assessment.* New York: Norton.

Nielsen, N.C. Jr., Hein, N., Reynolds, F.D., Miller, A.L., Karff, S.E., Cochran, A.C., & McLean, P. (Eds.). (1983). *Religions of the world.* New York: St. Martin's Press.

Orthner, D.K. (1986). *Pastoral counseling: Caring and caregivers in the United Methodist Church.* Nashville, TN: The General Board of Higher Education and Ministry of the United Methodist Church.

Oswald, R.M., & Kroeger, O. (1988). *Personality type and religious leadership.* Washington, DC: Alban Institute.

Randour, M.L. (Ed.). (1993). *Exploring sacred landscapes: Religious and spiritual experiences in psychotherapy.* New York: Columbia University Press.

Richardson, A., & Bowden, J. (1983). *The Westminster dictionary of christian theology.* Philadelphia: Westminster Press.

Smith, J.A. (Ed.). (1995). *The Harper Collins dictionary of religion.* San Francisco: Harper.

Stumpf, S.E. (1977). *Philosophy: History and problems.* New York: McGraw-Hill.

Thomas, H. (1965). *Biographical encyclopedia of philosophy.* Garden City: Doubleday.

Tucker, R.C. (Ed.). (1978). *The Marx-Engels reader* (2nd ed.). New York: Norton.

Weaver, A.J., Koenig, H.G., & Larson, D.B. (1997). Marriage and family therapists and the clergy: A need for clinical collaboration, training, and research. *Journal of Marital and Family Therapy, 23*(1), 13–25.

6

Strategic Marketing with Educators and the Educational Community

Complexity and diversity arise because the educational matrix has three aspects: developmental, multilevel, and political.

The complex systems and diversity in the educational field present a challenge to the mental health professional desiring to network or market products or services to educators. Complexity and diversity arise because the educational matrix has three aspects: developmental, multilevel, and political. Education is a continuous process for everyone at all stages of development, from preschoolers to adults taking continuing education classes. It is multilevel because it includes teachers, educational administrators, support staff, students, and parents of students as well as the local citizenry. A large percentage of the population is affected by or somehow involved in the educational matrix, and there are multiple theories/opinions about educational structure, methods, and philosophy. Diversity is a basic characteristic of educational theory and practice with advocates of various educational methods seldom being in agreement. The diversity may engender conflict between any of the constituencies involved with the educational system.

The educational matrix is also political. It involves politicians at all levels—local, state, and national—because the entire community has an investment in the process and outcome of the educational system. This civic component means that the local electorate votes on school board members, who then are responsible for the operation and effectiveness of the community educational system. In addition, state boards of education oversee the public schools and state colleges. The U.S. Department of Education also sets policies, standards, and procedures for public educational systems.

Taxpayers finance public education. Because the American public educational system is decentralized and controlled by the local community, there is no uniform federal school organization or curriculum. At its base, the American educational system includes two systems—the public and the private. In between the public and the private are hybrid systems such as the charter school. The private school system is further subdivided into nonsectarian and religious schools. These private educational systems may also have gender bifurcation. Each educational system has its particular philosophy and belief system. Knowing something of the rationale behind each system, or at minimum the system to which you may choose to market your products or services, will help you achieve success (see Recommended Reading).

Each educational system has its particular philosophy.

Due to local, state, and national involvement, teachers often are under a great deal of pressure and stress from each constituency. As a result, two national political action groups for teachers were formed: the National Education Association and the American Federation of Teachers (see Resources for addresses and web sites). These two groups focus on the working conditions, requirements, salary, class size, and other issues that affect educators and their ability to competently perform their job.

Teachers in private schools, on the other hand—from kindergarten through college—do not have to deal with as complex a system. They do not necessarily have to meet the same requirements. For example, private school teachers are not required to have licensure, but it is mandatory for teachers in the public school system.

As a mental health professional, a major element of your strategic planning and marketing process is to select specific educational constituencies for networking; then you must target points of entry. For example, decide whether to focus on the public or private schools within your locale. Then select a submarket (point of entry) for your first outreach effort such as parent-teacher associations, elementary school teachers, preschools and/or kindergartens, or guidance counselor associations. It is essential to be informed about the educational system dynamics within your locality. Patience and tenacity are required for success. Think strategically.

The Correlation of Psychology and Education

Johann Friedrich Herbart (1776–1841) is considered to be the founder of theoretical pedagogy. He incorporated metaphysics and psychology into the study of how people learn and established pedagogy as an autonomous science. He also attempted to give teaching a psychological rationale and highlighted student interest and spontaneity as elements of the learning process. For Herbart, ethics was the primary focus of education. The teacher's ultimate objective is character formation as the student develops an enlightened will and can make judgments regarding right and wrong.

During the late nineteenth century and early twentieth centuries, following on Herbart's ideas, educators made serious efforts to apply psychology to the art of teaching. In 1891, William James, first to develop an American psychology of education, initiated his psycho-physiological laboratory at Harvard University. According to James, the purpose of education was to organize the student's "powers of conduct so as to fit him to his social and physical environment. Interest must be awakened and broadened as the natural starting points of instruction" (Goetz, 1995, p. 67).

Another primary thinker was the American philosopher John Dewey. He and James both understood the human being as a living organism influenced by both heredity and environment. They were the first theorists to focus on the role of motivation and goal seeking in learning. Edward Lee Thorndike was another influential American figure in the field of educational psychology. He designed methods to measure and test children's intelligence and their ability to learn.

Freudians, too, had an effect on twentieth-century educational models. In the United States, the new psychologies greatly influenced educational theories and led to paradigm shifts in classroom teaching patterns. The former authoritarian models of transmission of knowledge were discontinuous with the newer understandings. These processes continue today as we hear calls from the public for a return to the "basics," while others call for educational programs that teach "how to think" instead of emphasizing a content orientation.

Two other early twentieth-century proponents of child-centered education are Francis W. Parker of the United States and Maria Montessori of Italy. Parker pioneered progressive education in the belief that child development was the proper focus of education. As superintendent of schools in Quincy, Massachusetts, he instituted programs incorporating physical activities, science, excursions, and creative self-expression through art, music, and crafts. His pedagogical style became known as the "Quincy method." By training teachers in his method, Parker furthered these early steps in formulating modern educational theory.

Montessori's basic premise was that the child needs freedom from parent and/or teacher domination. She directed her initial effort in educational reform toward enlightening the conscience of teachers so as to change the teacher-student paradigm. Teachers were not to assume a role of superiority but instead were to act as a kind director. Their task was to see that all went according to an overriding plan that facilitated children's mastery of skills needed for everyday life. Montessori attempted to create a frustration-free environment for the child. Her methods of early childhood education are now practiced worldwide in the Montessori schools.

Swiss psychologist Jean Piaget, using philosophical and psychological elements to study children's intellectual development, contributed greatly to educators' understanding of childhood capacities. Piaget posited that there are four stages in the development of intelligence:

1. From birth to 2 years, kinetic muscular intelligence develops.
2. From 2 to 7 or 8 years, learning and use of language enable symbolic thinking.
3. During the 8th through 12th years, the child masters concrete operations, and can understand classification, one-to-one correspondence, series, whole numbers, fractions, space, time, and chance. He or she begins to have some understanding of abstract ideas such as "responsibility" and can deal somewhat with mental symbols.
4. After the 12th year, ability develops to deal with formal mental processes that are not related to objects. The youth can begin to understand theories, and verbal teaching can now be used in a primary way.

As educational theories began to take on a scientific perspective, researchers began to incorporate philosophical and psychological principles into their models. This interaction between education and psychology continues today. There is a precedent, tradition, and history for mental health professionals to be involved with educators and the educational community. In the 1960s, the community mental health movement envisioned treating children in the schools with the hope that preventive psychiatry could promote mentally healthier adults and a healthier community life. Psychologists and psychiatrists were used as consultants to teachers about classroom issues (see Caplan, 1964).

Being informed and understanding this historical background will enhance your communication with educators and strengthen your connection with them. The history of the educational system is thoroughly covered in Dickson A. Mungazi's *Evolution of Educational Theory in the United States*; Paulo Freire's *Pedagogy of the Oppressed* is a good source for studying economic issues (see Recommended Reading). Be informed and creative! Think strategically!

Characteristics of Teachers

Of all teachers in the public elementary and secondary schools, 52 percent have a bachelor's degree and 42 percent have a master's degree; approximately 1 percent have a doctoral degree and 4.6 percent are education specialists (National Center for Education Statistics [NCES], Digest of Education Statistics web site, Table 67). They may have obtained their degrees at a college specializing in teacher training or a college or university that has an education degree program. Most programs include a teaching internship component and all states require licensing of all public school teachers, kindergarten through secondary school; licensing programs and requirements are infrequently reciprocal between states. There is a probationary teaching period, usually three years, after which a teacher may obtain tenure. Tenure means a teacher cannot be fired without a just cause and due process.

Most programs include a teaching internship component and all states require licensing of all public school teachers, kindergarten through secondary school; licensing programs and requirements are infrequently reciprocal between states.

Preschool teachers often have an associate's degree in early childhood development and/or in-service training programs related to child development. Teachers at the middle and secondary school levels often have master's degrees related to their field of expertise such as special education, library sciences, or curriculum development. Principals and administrators frequently have a master's degree and many have obtained doctorates related to school administration. Vocational teachers and adult education teachers often possess expertise in the field (e.g., electrical, plumbing, culinary arts) as well as degreed credentials.

There are over 30,000 school districts in the United States and 2,561,294 teachers in public elementary and secondary schools. Nearly three-fourths are women and their median age is 46. Of teachers, 76 percent are married. There are 378,365 teachers in private elementary and secondary schools and 285,235 are female, with the majority being in the 40 to 49 age group. Like the public school system, minorities comprise a fraction of the teaching staff (NCES, *Digest of Education Statistics*, Tables 67 and 69).

There are over 30,000 school districts in the United States and 2,561,294 teachers in public elementary and secondary schools.

The average number of hours in the required school day are 7.3, and elementary teachers spend an average of 47 hours per week on all teaching duties; secondary teachers spend an average of 52 hours. The average number of teaching days in the school year is 180. Most teachers have 10-month contracts with a 2-month vacation period during the summer. Teachers often use this time for continuing education events.

Although there is wide variation among the states, average salaries for full-time teachers in public elementary and secondary schools with approximately 15 years experience is a base of $36,182 for men and $33,384 for women. The average base salary for first-year teachers is $23,544. Private school teachers with 15 years experience make considerably less with $26,120 being the base for men and $20,669 for women. The base salaries in both the public and private school systems may be increased by taking on additional responsibilities. Preschool teachers are the lowest paid, with 40 percent making between $12,000 and $18,000 per year. College and university faculty have an average salary of $51,000 per year (NCES, *Digest of Education Statistics,* Table 73).

Throughout the school years, teachers play an important role in children's development. The teacher-student interaction can shape the young child's view of self in the world and affect educational success or failure. Kindergarten and elementary school teachers use many hands-on skills involving artwork, music, audiovisuals, computers, and other tools when they introduce children to the basics of language, numbers, social studies, and the sciences.

Secondary school teachers build on basic skills for moving more deeply into the subject matter and its relationship to the student's world. Youths are prepared for entering higher academic levels and/or the world of work. Secondary school teachers often specialize in particular fields such as language arts, history, languages, mathematics, biology, or chemistry.

Teachers may have responsibility for one classroom and/or participate in some form of team-teaching modality. In the major urban areas, they likely will have a multiethnic class composition. They often must prepare classroom curriculum and presentations to match the needs and abilities of a heterogeneous grouping of students. (Private school teachers may have a more homogeneous group.) Since teachers now use considerable technology in teaching, they must continually update teaching skills.

Teachers have complex, demanding responsibilities and interpersonal interactions:

> They plan, evaluate and assign lessons; prepare, administer, and grade tests; listen to oral presentations; and maintain classroom discipline. They observe and evaluate a student's performance and potential, and increasingly use new assessment methods. . . . Teachers also grade papers, prepare report cards, and meet with parents and school staff . . . teachers oversee study halls and homerooms and supervise extracurricular activities. They identify physical or mental problems and refer students to the proper resource or agency for diagnosis and treatment. Secondary school teachers occasionally assist students in choosing courses, colleges, and careers. Teachers also participate in education conferences and workshops. ("School Teachers—Kindergarten, Elementary, and Secondary"; 1998–1999 *Occupational Outlook Handbook*. Bureau of Labor Statistics web site, http://stats.bls.gov/oes/oes_data.htm)

Understanding the demographics as well as the overall system in education can help you put things into perspective and enable you to generate new ideas, pinpoint weaknesses, or see new trends.

Marketplace

Our complex and diverse educational system daily touches millions of people.

Our complex and diverse educational system touches millions of people daily. Now that education is understood as a lifelong learning process, the market is growing. In 1994, there were 4,904,757 people employed in the U.S. public school system (kindergarten through high school). The number of students was 44,111,000. In the private school systems, first grade through high school, the 1993–1994 data indicated that there were 534,636 people employed throughout the United States. The estimated number of students was 5,596,000 (NCES, *Digest of Education Statistics,* Table 60). In the fall of 1997, there were a total of 74,100,000 students at all levels of the educational system including public and private schools (NCES, *Digest of Education Statistics,* Table 1).

Consider the number of parents and other community members involved with these students. If you choose to network with the education community and patiently build relationships with your selected niche market, your practice could flourish for many years. The market potential is great.

Future

The student body is projected to grow approximately 1 percent to 2 percent a year through 2005 with a total student body of 60,544,000 projected for the public primary and secondary schools and 9,510,000 for the private primary and secondary schools (NCES, *Digest of Education Statistics*, Table 2). New schools and additional teachers will be needed. Congress recently voted funding for the building of new schools and the hiring of 100,000 additional teachers to achieve a smaller teacher-student ratio. The projected number of teachers needed in 2005 is 3,339,000. Of this number, 2,918,000 will be needed in the public schools and 420,000 in the private schools. The educational system will be a growth industry for the next several decades, particularly because the adult education market also is growing. And, as mentioned earlier, the numbers in the educational matrix are even higher if one includes the parents and community organizations that are adjuncts to the educational system. With these projections in mind, you need to consider the long-term investment potential of offering services/products to the education market.

The student body is projected to grow approximately 1% to 2% a year through 2,005 with a total student body of 60,544,000 projected for the public primary and secondary schools and 9,510,000 for the private primary and secondary schools.

The Needs of the Educational Community

Since the educational community includes various constituencies, we will briefly consider needs of three major groups: teachers, students, the general public.

Teachers Point to Their Needs

Studying the needs of your target audience can help you market your services. Pinpointing their stated weaknesses or finding areas where they need assistance will enable you to focus on the appropriate product to achieve the best results. Research is always key to discovering your market's needs.

Research is always key to discovering your market's needs.

In a survey conducted by the U.S. Department of Education in 1993–1994, public elementary school teachers cited the following as the top five serious problems in their schools (NCES, *Digest of Education Statistics*, Table 27):

1. Students come unprepared to learn (24.3 percent).
2. Lack of parental involvement (23 percent).
3. Poverty (20.8 percent).
4. Student apathy (15.6 percent).
5. Student disrespect for teachers (15.3 percent).

Private elementary school teachers cited few problems; the highest problem area was lack of parental involvement (2.8 percent).

Secondary teachers in public school systems, cited these serious problems:

- Student apathy (38 percent).
- Students come unprepared to learn (36 percent).
- Lack of parental involvement (34.5 percent).
- Student absenteeism (27.1 percent).
- Student disrespect for teachers (23.6 percent).
- Student use of alcohol (23.1 percent).

Private school secondary teachers cited the following serious problems:

- Student use of alcohol (11 percent).
- Student apathy (9.7 percent).

In a 1993–1994 survey, public and private school elementary and secondary school teachers shared many perceptions about teaching and school conditions (NCES, *Digest of Education Statistics,* Table 28). The information from the survey indicated that there are major systemic differences between public and private school settings, other than in the area of salary. Public school teachers did not feel as supported or appreciated in their work as private school teachers. Marketing strategies would therefore need to be different for teachers in the two different settings.

Students Point to Their Needs

Often, the issues that teachers consider most pressing are quite different from those perceived by the students. Another way to market your services is to also include areas of interest that greatly concern the student body. Therefore, you should be aware of students' problems as well as those of the teachers. For students in Grades 7–12, a 1996 Harris Poll indicated the following serious problems (NCES, *Digest of Education Statistics*, Table 15.1):

- Gang violence (26 percent).
- Physical fights between members of different groups of friends (26 percent).
- Hostile or threatening remarks between groups of students (25 percent).
- Threats or destructive acts, other than physical fights (24 percent).
- Turf battles between different groups of students (21 percent).

Percentages for these issues were even higher among urban students (e.g., gang violence, 36 percent; physical fights, 33 percent; turf battles between different groups of students, 30 percent). When race and ethnicity further differentiated the survey, the percentages were higher for African American and Hispanic students in all five categories. Think about your background and how you can best relate to the education system. Perhaps you have experience in working with anger, hostility, and violence in children or work with cases of domestic abuse. In any event, these concerns of students could be avenues for you to approach educators and to offer your services.

Think about your background and how you can best relate to the education system.

Another survey invited the students to grade the teaching skills of their teachers. While 77 percent of the students gave their teachers an "A" or "B" for understanding the subjects they teach, only 39 percent gave them an "A" or "B" for making learning interesting for everyone and only 27 percent gave them a similar grade for taking an interest in students' home and personal lives. (NCES, *Digest of Education Statistics*, Table 75.) These areas could be starting points for creating workshops that address communication between students and teachers.

These latter statistics could correlate to teachers' concerns about student apathy, absenteeism, and students' concerns about violence potentials at school. In the area of encouraging students' academic interest, 61 percent of Caucasian students graded their teachers "A" or "B," while only 42 percent of African American students did so and only 44 percent of Hispanic students graded teachers "A" or "B" on the statement.

Overall, 57 percent of students felt the quality of teachers was "pretty good," 20 percent felt it was "only fair," and 16 percent felt teacher quality was "excellent."

The data point to differences between what teachers and students see as serious concerns. Try to correlate such data in the development and marketing of your products and services. If you are trained in multicultural and diversity issues, you could offer workshops for teachers about empowering students from particular ethnic communities. You could also offer workshops for students around communication and assertion skills.

If you are trained in multicultural and diversity issues, you could offer workshops for teachers about empowering students from particular ethnic communities.

The Public Points to Their Needs

Data based on Gallup Polls show that the general public thinks the following are major problems faced by public schools in 1996 (NCES, *Digest of Education Statistics,* Table 23):

- Use of drugs (16 percent).
- Lack of discipline (15 percent).
- Fighting/violence/gangs (14 percent).
- Lack of financial support (13 percent).

The perception of the public differs from that of the teachers, as indicated in the following statistics:

- Lack of respect (2 percent).
- Lack of family structure/problems of home life (4 percent).
- Pupil's lack of interest/truancy (3 percent).
- Large schools/overcrowding (8 percent).

These percentages point to disparities in perceptions between teachers, students, and the public about the needs of the educational community. Numerous variables can contribute to such differences. However, the variances are likely to reflect inadequate communication between the respective groups and lack of knowledge about the differing populations and divergent experiences within the educational community. If you are trained in forming dialogue groups and forums, you can develop several services/products related to the feedback and input from those related to the educational system.

By visualizing the constituencies in the educational community, and knowing their needs, you will find a wide range of possibilities for developing a niche market.

Competitors

As you begin to connect with those in the educational professions, ask them about other mental health professionals with whom they work. Obtain names, addresses, and telephone numbers as well as any written material that may be available about their services, products, and fee structures. Contact these colleagues and schedule a meeting or invite them to an open house at your office. Discuss possibilities around cooperation and ask them to fill out a Resource Directory Worksheet describing their skills and areas of expertise.

As you begin to connect with those in the educational professions, ask them about other mental health professionals with whom they work.

Use the Yellow Pages to locate guidance, career, and vocational counselors, school psychologists, and other counselors/therapists who may focus on school and education issues. Check also for associations of these professions, such as your state school psychologists' association. Obtain a mailing list from them for school psychologists in your area. Mail them your materials, along with a Resource Directory Worksheet to be returned to you. Follow up with a telephone call and an invitation to meet.

The Story of Your Educational Experiences

The mixed bag of your educational experiences can make this milieu problematic by easily evoking power and authority issues. Mental health professionals who enter the educational markets must confront their educational past. Dealing with this past is essential to success in the market. As you consider points of entry and reflect on the mindmap (Figure 6.1) depiction of points of entry, be attentive to your inner process and allow the input to assist you in choosing where to begin your outreach to the educational community.

Mental health professionals who enter the educational markets must confront their educational past. Dealing with this past is essential to success in the market.

You can facilitate this process by reviewing your family-of-origin genogram. Ask yourself the following questions as you take a family educational history. If you don't know answers to the questions, become the family investigator and seek out answers:

- Are there any teachers in the family? Are any family members employed by the school system? What is their input to other family members regarding their work and the system?
- What has been the family response to their vocation?
- What educational levels have been attained by family members? Did they attend public or private schools? If private, was it religious or nonsectarian?
- What has been shared about their experience? What was the quality of the experience?
- What has been your educational experience from kindergarten through graduate school? Your siblings? How do you rate it?
- Who were your favorite teachers? Worst teachers? In your experience and/or perceptions, what were the characteristics of each that made them "good" or "bad" teachers? As you reflect on these relationships, what are you feeling now?
- What are your family's belief systems, biases, prejudices, regarding education and the educational system (school taxes, the school board, election of board members)?
- Did any family members ever serve on the school board?
- What is your trust level of teachers?
- Do you have special training that would correlate with the experiences and needs of educational professionals?
- Do you have children in school? If so, public or private? How do you make decisions regarding your children's education?
- Other questions.

Take time for honest self-evaluation and reflection on the preceding questions, and make sure that you respect and feel comfortable working with the educational professional community. As appropriate, share your educational experiences in a manner that will aid bridge building with the educational community. Allow your educational history and personal experience to be a guide in selecting points of entry. If you have had a private secular school education, you may choose to focus your services and products to that community. Similarly, if you have had a parochial school education or a public school education, you will have other experiences to draw on in building relationships.

Niche Experience

Evaluate your training and experience and the types of clients you most often work with. The self-evaluation may expose areas to where you could seek further education and/or specialized training, but focus your outreach on the foundation you currently have. If you have received training in family systems therapy, you may focus your networking with the parent-teachers organization and other family-oriented organizations that relate to the schools. You could also direct it to guidance counselors and school psychologists. If you have training in vocational counseling and the use of an instrument such as the Meyers-Briggs Type Indicator, you may choose to focus your marketing to teachers, guidance counselors, and parents of 11th and 12th graders. If you have training in working with young children, then you may connect with directors of day-care centers and preschools, school principals, teachers, and the PTO in elementary schools. If your specialty is trauma or eating disorders, you may want to connect with school nurses. Use your knowledge and training in communication skills to develop workshops for educators around professional communication—teachers frequently hold conferences with parents and often are involved in team-teaching.

No matter where you select your point of entry, you must allow time for building a relationship with the participants. Think systemically (e.g., teachers, parents, students, and greater community). The educational matrix is large and offering your services as a specialist as well as a general practitioner will expand your possibilities and potentials. As a general practitioner, you have many skills to share:

No matter where you select your point of entry, you must allow time for building a relationship with the participants.

- Knowledge about working with people in crisis or trauma.
- Assistance with life transitions—job changes, injuries and illness, separations and divorces, grief and loss.
- Clinical issues such as depression, anxiety, and personality disorders.
- Children, adolescents, and young adult concerns.
- Communication skills training.
- Interviewing, evaluation, assessment, and intervention models.
- Knowledge of developmental models.
- Resourcing/referring to specialists.

In addition to the preceding possibilities, you may want to develop other services or products. Marketing to the educational community can require a plan that spans several years. Some of the following possibilities may require further continuing education and/or credentialing. As you strategize your marketing potential, consider these following specific niche areas as components that could very well be applicable to a continuing professional development plan.

School-Based Consulting. It has long been recognized that integrating mental health and educational programs could be highly beneficial to children, adolescents, their families, and the wider community (see Resources). One private practitioner has developed a model for school-based consulting and trains mental health professionals interested in a school-based consulting practice called "School-Based Collaboration with Families." He uses a systemic model, which includes the child, parents, extended family, teachers, and administrators in the interventions and outcome. He calls this process collaborative team intervention. He has published a book describing the specialty (O'Callaghan, 1993) and offers telephone supervision to school personnel. Contact him to learn more about his program and training opportunities (see Resources).

Eating Disorders. Eating disorders are frequently manifested in younger girls. A recent book (Bode, 1998) based on a survey of 100 Long Island, New York, eighth graders found that 12 percent had forced themselves to vomit and half of them had been on at least one program of weight loss. A November 27, 1998, *Boston Globe* feature on preadolescents shared the findings of Dr. Timothy Brewerton, Professor of Psychiatry and Behavioral Sciences and the Director of the Eating Disorders Program at Medical University of South Carolina. He conducted a 1993 survey with two colleagues. Out of 3,175 students in Grades 5 through 8, he found the following:

- 42 percent wanted to lose weight.
- 31.4 percent had dieted.
- 4.8 percent had induced vomiting.
- 2.4 percent had taken diet pills.
- 3 percent had used diuretics or laxatives to lose weight.

Developing a school-based program or in-office group for these particular ages would meet a need. Cofacilitating the group with a school nurse would be helpful in marketing your service to the community.

Developing a school-based program or in-office group for these particular ages would meet a need.

Marketing to Learning Centers. Parents of preadolescents and teens who enroll their children in these programs are motivated and committed to their child's success in school. Share with the director of the learning centers how your expertise in emotional problems correlates with learning difficulties and how your services can be mutually enhancing. Suggest a mutual referral system. Offer to copresent with the learning center at informational meetings. Distribute your marketing materials.

Marketing to Licensed Day-Care Providers. If you want to work with young children and their families, this has potential for a niche market. Contact the State Office of Child Care Services (in your state the office may have a different title). They will be able to direct you to licensed day-care providers in your region as well as educational and in-service training coordinators. You can then develop your strategies, products, and services to this particular niche. It is a rapidly growing market.

Facilitating Peer Support Groups for New Teachers. Facing a classroom of anywhere from 18 to 30 children can be overwhelming for the first-time teacher. Building a relationship with an experienced teacher and codeveloping and facilitating monthly group meetings for new teachers would fill an important need. The group, consisting of 8 to 10 members, could meet monthly from August through June for 90 minutes.

Developing Presentations and Workshops around a National Observance Day (see Resources for more complete list). For example, American Education Week, sponsored by the National Education Association (NEA), is usually in November and has a yearly theme. The 1998 theme was "Teaching Children to Think and Dream." The NEA web site has numerous suggestions and resources for activities during the week. You could:

- Prepare and offer a workshop around the theme to local PTOs.
- Prepare an in-service training for educators on the theme.
- Offer workshop around theme at statewide annual teachers conference.

Workshops/Presentations for Students. Offer workshops to religious schools, congregations, youth groups; public school clubs; scouting groups, and so on. There are many resources around developing programs that focus on life skills and relationships (see Resources). Follow your interests and abilities.

Network with Your Local State-Funded Parent Education Programs. For example, Massachusetts has community-based family network and/or family resource coalitions/collaborations. These groups sponsor several skills-building and parenting support programs for families with children, from infancy to high school, and other services such as providing free museum passes. Offer to provide a program based on your areas of interest and ability.

Additional Niche Programs and Services (add your own ideas, related to your local community and its needs).

- Attention-Deficit Hyperactivity Disorder.
- Parenting children with chronic illness.
- Parenting children who are developmentally disabled.
- Parenting intellectually gifted children.
- Gifts and challenges of single parenting.
- Children with impulse disorders.
- Helping children and teens learn anger management.
- Parenting and multiple birth issues.
- Signs of and treatment for depression in children or youth.
- Developing resiliency in children.
- Children and stress.
- Relationship skills for teens.
- Team-building for teachers.

The mental health professional brings a wealth of knowledge and ability to the educational field and often has experience working with most of the age groups in this market.

The mental health professional brings a wealth of knowledge and ability to the educational field and often has experience working with most of the age groups in this market. You know how important educational experiences are in supporting self-esteem, personal development, and interpersonal skills. You also recognize the potential here for intervention and treatment. Nurture this mindset as you develop brochures and letters for constituencies within the educational system (see Figures 6.3, 6.4 through 6.7).

Engaging the Marketplace

Your experiences and transferable skills will help you move forward in developing your products and services for the educational community.

Point of Entry

Instead of taking a hit-or-miss approach, select a point of entry into the educational matrix. Deciding where to begin offering your services/products (your point of entry) is responsive to the multiple systems within the educational community. There are multiple entry points into the system, especially in the field of public education, which involves political constituencies and publicly elected school boards. Use your time and money carefully; the educational pond is large and deep.

Whether you choose one, or more than one, point of entry, include relationship-building time in your outreach efforts. In marketing to educational professionals and the educational community, trust levels are prerequisite and will increase the marketing time commitment. In selecting your point of entry, be attentive to the extent of personal and professional resources necessary for success.

Prudent strategizing and marketing will include:

- Becoming familiar with the educational systems in your location.
- Becoming well informed about the local educational issues.
- Studiously and prudently selecting your point of entry based on where you feel the most capable and the most resonant.
- Using point of entry for strategizing your market, products, and services.
- Focusing on your local community.
- Reviewing your mindmap as to potential entry points. Any entity on the mindmap may provide your initial direction. Construct a mindmap for each outreach program you develop.

Construct a mindmap for each outreach program you develop.

Choosing one or two points of entry involves self-reflection and practice evaluation. Practice evaluation includes:

- *The size of your practice.* Are you a solo practitioner or are you involved in a small or large group practice? If you are a solo practitioner, do you have adequate backup and referral resources available to you for possible psychological and pharmacological evaluations? Are you networked with community resources for families and children? Are you prepared to deal with multiproblem families?
- *Fees.* Are you on managed-care and/or insurance panels? Are you approved for Medicare? Do you have a sliding fee scale? Be up front about your fee schedule when communicating with educators and the education community.
- *Credentials.* Are you licensed? This will be an important criterion for referral consideration within the education matrix. If not licensed, are you a member of any recognized national professional groups? For example, not all states have licensed marriage and family therapists, but it is possible to be a clinical member of the American Association of Marriage and Family Therapists.
- *Knowledge about the local educational community.* Consider doing an "Information Interview" with educators and other leaders in the education community about their particular needs and what you, as a mental health professional, might be able to offer or resource to fill such needs. An information interview would include questions about the composition of the group or school; its culture/ethnicity; what's going well; where assistance could be used, and so on.

Finding Contacts

Ask your peers and other professional colleagues for names of any educators they know or have worked with and would recommend as a potential resource.

First, get in touch with the people you already know in the education field—from licensed day-care providers to university professors. Ask these men and women to recommend educators they may know in your locality related to your point of entry. Ask your peers and other professional colleagues for names of any educators they know or have worked with and would recommend as a potential resource. Ask your friends and neighbors. As you begin to collect names, ask permission to use their name in your introductory letter. When there is a telephone contact with the educator or member of the education community, use that person's name. Recommendations from a reputable, known individual help greatly in strategic marketing and building networks.

If you have no recommendations from an individual, name the referral resource you have used to make contact—telephone directory or Yellow Pages, Internet, and so on. Just as we are interested in how clients or contacts have learned of our services, so are other professionals.

Telephone Book/Business Pages/Yellow Pages. Telephone books are a rich resource as you begin putting together a marketing plan. The Yellow Pages not only lists all the private schools, nursery through university, it also contains listings for resources such as guidance counselors, vocational counselors, and career counselors. Public schools are found in the city and/or state listings of your telephone book. Use this information to refine and/or define your point of entry. If your community has a religion-based elementary school and you have decided that you want to market your products to educators affiliated with a religious community, then you may well have located your first point of entry.

State Education Directory. Contact the offices of your state department of education and request a copy of the *State Education Directory.* This provides a wealth of information regarding school districts, schools, personnel, and so on. This is a primary resource that you will use again and again.

State Teachers Associations. The state teachers' associations are found in the business pages along with your state federation of teachers. Call or write the state teachers' associations and state federation of teachers group and ask for their calendar of events, particularly annual conference dates, meeting dates, and contact people in your local area. National associations of teachers and the PTO have web sites with links to the state and local organizations (see Resources). Inquire about having a booth at annual meetings and ask whether they produce a newsletter. If they answer "yes" about a newsletter, ask for a rate sheet.

Call or write the state teacher's associations and state federation of teachers group and ask for their calendar of events, particularly annual conference dates, meeting dates, and contact people in your local area.

Education Special Interest Groups. Ask the teachers' groups how they are organized (e.g., committees). Obtain a list and see if you have collegial interests with a particular group; for example, a committee that deals with multicultural and diversity issues in the classroom. If you have an interest in such an area or have expertise in the field, contact the committee and inquire about collaborating on a project. You might develop and colead a workshop at an annual meeting.

You will want this type of information to develop your mailing list and to focus your interests. Networking with a committee and/or group with mutual interests is a good point of entry. Call the chair of the committee, share your background and interest, ask for meeting dates, and request a mailing list of committee members. Next survey the list for any names you know and share it with colleagues, friends, or family to see if they know any teachers on the list. Begin with those where an introduction by letter or telephone may be possible.

The local school and/or school board may also have committees dealing with special issues that interest you. When you arrange a meeting with the principal or superintendent, this would be an area to ask about. Find the name of the chairperson or coordinator and contact that person. Write an introductory letter and mail it with your brochure. Call the person within five business days following their receipt of the letter and arrange a meeting to discuss your mutual interests and how you may be helpful to one another.

School Counselors Directory. The Massachusetts School Counselors Association publishes a directory of all members once a year. Locate the school counselors association for your state and inquire as to their directory, regularly scheduled meetings, and newsletters. Locate the school counselors in your district or region and mail them your brochure and resource information sheet. Call those who respond and arrange an introductory meeting. If no one responds, call anyway. They are busy, and it is worth the effort.

Contact a local, public or private, elementary, middle, or secondary school, and ask for the name, address, and telephone number of the president of their parent-teachers organization.

Parent-Teachers Organization/Association. Contact a local, public or private, elementary, middle, or secondary school, and ask for the name, address, and telephone number of the president of their parent-teachers organization. Write a letter of introduction and mail it, along with your brochure, to the president. Call within five days to arrange a meeting or telephone interview. Ask about the needs of the local school, PTA, and students. Volunteer as a speaker for one of their meetings. Ask the president for the name, telephone number, and address of the state PTA president and make contact there also. Ask about dates of annual meetings, availability of booth space, and workshop possibilities.

The Internet. For those of you who have computers and are online or have access to online resources, there are hundreds, if not thousands, of excellent resources, including government organizations, related to education. Individual Internet sites may contain subcommittees with names and addresses of members with their addresses and telephone numbers. It may also offer links to other related sites. Online resources tend to be friendly and responsive (see Resources).

Marketing Plan

After you have completed your review and gathered information about the educational community, develop a mindmap to represent the potentials and possibilities for connecting with and marketing to the educational matrix. List your resources in this market. Make use of your networking system in your marketing strategy.

The mindmap presents the information streams and connections that reflect your particular interests and specialties.

The mindmap presents the information streams and connections that reflect your particular interests and specialties. It will be the guide for your point-of-entry strategizing. You may return to it again and again as you develop your short- and long-term marketing strategy. It is helpful to develop a mindmap for each point of entry you select (see Figure 6.1).

Having done the mindmap, you now move to the next phase, which is to develop your Goal-Setting Worksheet. It is helpful to develop a goal sheet for each point of entry you select (see Figure 6.2).

Services and Products

Review educators' needs as well as your niche experience to develop services and products for the education community. The location for providing your offerings could be the school, your office, and/or other community settings. These could also be presented as in-service training events or presentations. Use your imagination and creativity. Several of the following suggestions could be developed as workshops for conferences.

- Communication skills—
  - Active listening skills.
  - Reading body language.
  - Emotional cues.

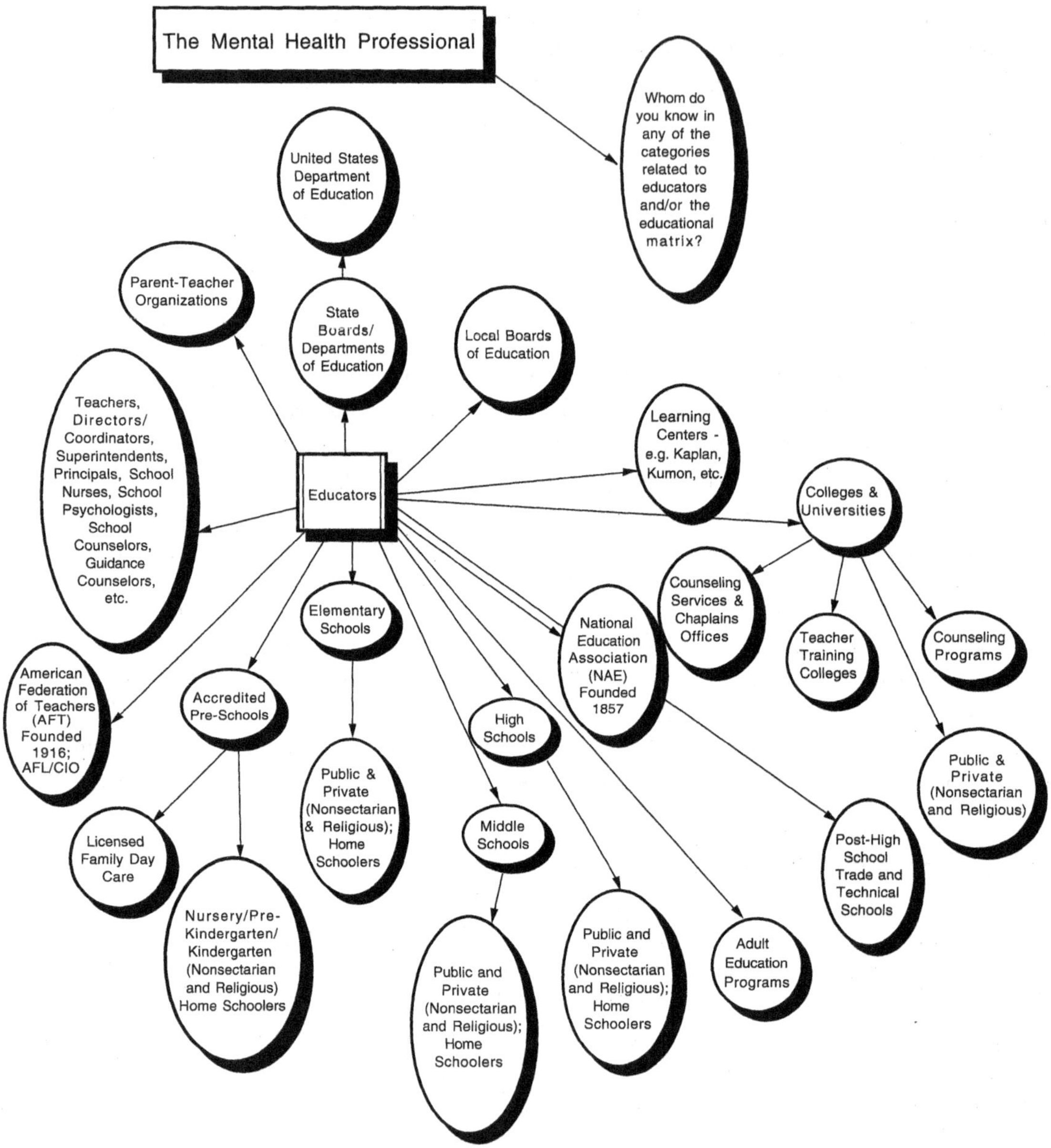

FIGURE 6.1 Mindmap—Educators and the Education Community

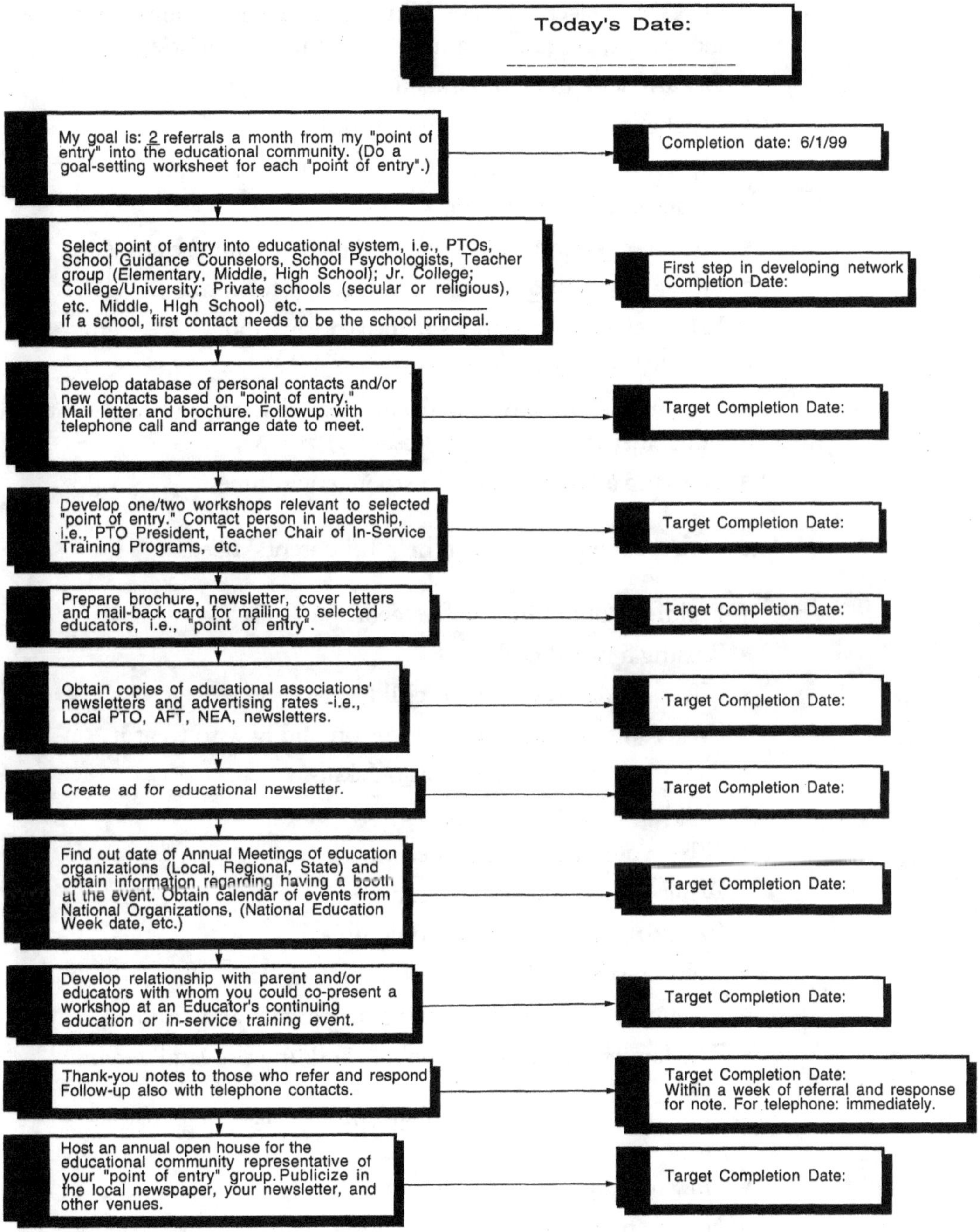

FIGURE 6.2 Educators Goal-Setting Worksheet

- Stress management (breathing, meditation, time management, movement, guided imaging, establishing boundaries, etc.).
- Dealing with difficult students.
- Teacher-parent communication skills.
- Myers-Briggs Type Indicators and teaching.
- Mediation skills training.
- Effects of parental divorce and remarriage on the student.
- Preventing burnout in the teaching profession.
- Issues related to teacher's identity formation.
- Establishing appropriate boundaries.
- Dynamics of healthy and dysfunctional systems (families, organizations, institutions, businesses, etc.).
- Creating a harmonious classroom environment.

These are areas where you can help fill parents' needs:

- Building your child's self-esteem.
- Raising a moral child.
- Effects of divorce on your children.
- Symptoms of childhood depression and how to treat it.
- Parent-teacher communication skills.
- Helping your child succeed at school.
- What your gifted child needs.
- What your special child needs.
- Parenting a child with chronic illness.
- Helping your child make and keep friends.
- Communication skill-building for parents and children.
- The family meeting—A tool for building the family team.

These are areas where you can help fill the needs of adolescents:

- How to deal with conflict.
- How to negotiate and compromise—family, school, friends, and job.

- Becoming a peer leader.
- Saying "no" without losing friends.
- Communicating with parents and teachers.
- Myers-Briggs Type Indicator for teenagers.
- National screening days—adolescent depression, anxiety, eating disorders (select a setting where teens feel comfortable).
- Learning about your study style and enhancing study skills.
- Make a presentation to a health or marriage and family class at the private or public high school.
- Have a booth at the middle and high school career day event.
- Offer individual vocational and career counseling if you have expertise with any testing instruments geared to these areas.

Continuing Education Programs and/or In-Service Training

Developing workshops or presentations for continuing education and/or in-service training is a helpful way to build a network with educators. Contact the chair for the continuing education committee of the teachers' association (at the local and state level) and ask to be added to the mailing list. Inquire about the programs they've had over the past one or two years, what the attendance has been, the procedures for developing and offering a continuing education event, and how much lead time is required. Share your areas of interest and specialty and ascertain whether any events have focused on that area. Coleading such a workshop or presentation with an educator or other individual related to the educational community offers strong potential for marketing your service or product.

In-service training is often offered at the school where the educator is employed. Contact the teacher who coordinates such offerings and inquire about their needs, ascertaining if there is a match with your areas of expertise, and offer to present a workshop. Always take your marketing materials for distribution.

Look for those with whom you have similar interests and like-mindedness regarding your areas of interest.

Coleading Workshops with a Teacher and/or Parent and/or Adolescent. As you begin to make connections with educators and others in the education community you will uncover relationship possibilities. Look for those with whom you have similar interests and like-mindedness regarding your areas of interest. Explore with them possibilities of developing a product or program. You may cofacilitate workshops or panel discussions around topics of mutual interest and expertise. Here are some suggestions:

- Attention deficit disorder.
- Behavior modification in the classroom—teachers and parents working together.
- Diversity of student learning styles.
- Myers-Briggs Type Indicator—a tool for the teacher, parent, and student.
- Students and divorce—what to look for.
- Parenting children with disabilities.
- Communication skills for adolescents.
- Peer counseling and adolescents—positive support.
- Eating disorders and the adolescent female.

Develop a Mutual Referral System with School Psychologists, Guidance Counselors, Vocational Counselors, and College Counselors. Just as you refer to other professionals when your client's needs involve an area in which you do not have expertise, so sometimes a need may arise for an evaluation requiring specialized psychological testing, vocational, and/or career counseling. As you begin to build a relationship with education professionals, you may use them as a referral resource (always give clients more than one name). Referring to such specialists may well result in your beginning to receive referrals from them. This could also provide an avenue for building a relationship with an education specialist with whom you would colead workshops. Use the Resource Directory Worksheet to begin networking with school psychologists, guidance counselors, and career counselors (see below). It will be included with your initial mailing to selected education professionals.

As you begin to build a relationship with education professionals, you may use them as a referral resource.

Trade Shows and Conferences (PTO, Teachers' Association, Guidance Counselors Association). These events provide important venues for networking with and marketing your services and products to those in the educational community. Contact your local and state PTO representatives, teacher associations, and guidance counselors association for dates of their annual meetings and arrange to rent a booth or table if they are available. Have the following items for display and distribution (include any products or services that would be pertinent to the education community):

- *Brochures.* Your brochure, including a basic one as well as brochures or flyers highlighting your niche areas. You may also use a brochure describing your particular field, for example, marriage and family therapy. These can often be obtained in bulk through your professional association. Be sure to have your name, address, and telephone number on the brochure.
- *Business card.* Your business card and other inexpensive handouts with your name, office address, and telephone number (writing pens, note pads).
- *Flyers.* Describing your workshop topics and dates.
- *Sign-in sheet.* Have a space for name, address, and telephone number. Follow up with a letter thanking them for stopping by your booth.

Having done your prior work in considering the point of entry with which you choose to begin marketing your services and products, now select the specialty, subspecialty, or special interest groups where you want to offer your services or products. Develop your brochures around your specialties and niche areas, create other enclosures, and proceed.

Outreach Vehicles

Outreach vehicles increase your visibility in your target professional grouping. Examples of the necessary pieces are given on the next several pages. Adapt them to reflect your location and your expertise. Figure 6.3 shows a sample brochure. Most educational professionals, as do other professionals, prefer cooperation and harmony. Write your letters with these qualities in mind. Keep all correspondence to a single page. Name your referral source and niche specialty. Figures 6.4 through 6.7 show examples of letters relative to several situations and can be easily adapted for different educator and/or school populations.

The Alpha Centr offers psychoeducation, counseling, consultation and assistance with locating needed resources. We are sensitive to and respectful of personal confidentiality..

Call 781.322.3051 for

Family & Child Counseling
By exploring relationship patterns, the family may develop healthier styles of relating and dealing with problems.

Couples Counseling
Couples are assisted in clarifying their hopes and expectations of the relationship, enhancing communication skills, and co-creating the type of relationship they desire.

Individual Counseling and Personal Growth
By considering interpersonal behaviors in your relationships and work experiences, and gaining awareness of your relational style and goals, new options and resources may be developed.

Separation Counseling and/or Divorce Mediation
When a relationship must end, impartial caring mediation can help you take charge of arrangements, avoid unnecessary injury to spouses and children, and save an average of 90% of the cost of litigated divorce.

Consultation
If you are wondering what to do about a situation and would like an objective viewpoint and/or resources or referrals, we will work with you in accomplishing your goals.

In-Service Trainings, Continuing Education Events
We will team with you in planning and facilitating a program and process which will forward your goals for a successful group experience.

The Alpha Centre

Sliding Fee Scale available for Uninsured and Private Pay Clients

Accessible by Public Transportation (Take the Bus or The Orange Line to Malden Center)

Parking Available On-street and in Parking Garages or Parking Lots

Elevator Building
Handicap Accessible

Directions by car to Malden:

Rt. 60 East to Main Street; turn left onto Main Street and take the second left onto Pleasant Street; 6 Pleasant Street is at the corner of Main and Pleasant Street

The Alpha Centre
6 Pleasant St. Ste. 214
Malden MA 02148

Phone: 781.322.5051
Fax: 781.662.8575

It is a sign of wisdom, not weakness, to ask for help.

The Alpha Centre

.....a resource for educators and the education community

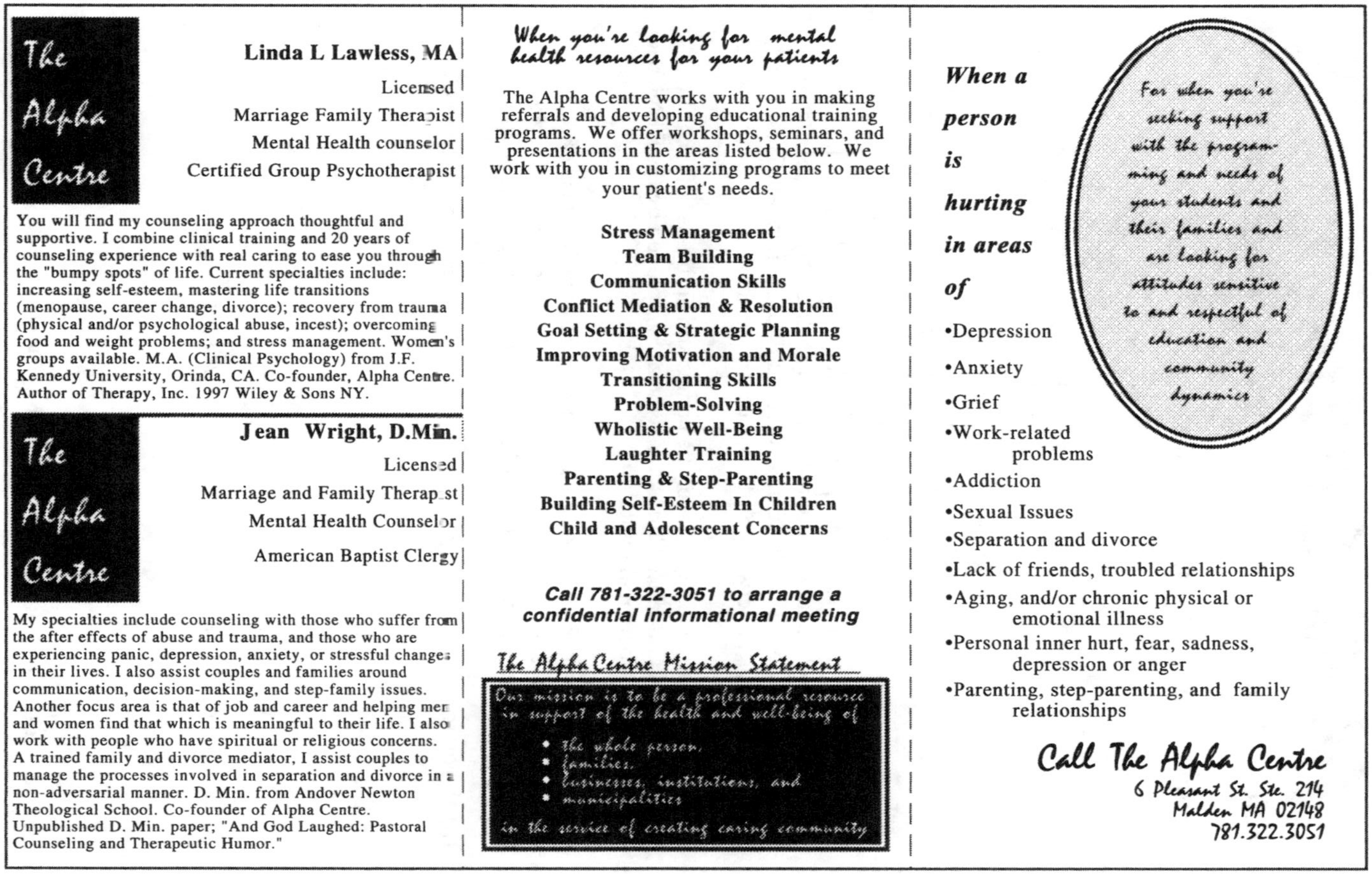

FIGURE 6.3 Sample Brochure for Educators

Alpha Centre

6 Pleasant Street Suite 214 Malden MA 02148 617-322-3051

Our mission is to be a professional resource in support of the health and well-being of
- The whole person
- Families
- Businesses, institutions, and
- Municipalities

in the service of creating caring community

Our services include psychoeducational workshops on:

IDENTIFYING CHILDREN WITH MENTAL HEALTH ISSUES

BUILDING SELF-ESTEEM IN CHILDREN & TEENS

TEAM BUILDING FOR EDUCATORS

TEACHER-PARENT COMMUNICATION

PERSONALITY TYPE & THE TEACHER

MEDITATION FOR TEENS

RAISING A MORAL CHILD

HOW TO MOTIVATE STUDENTS

DIVERSITY OF LEARNING STYLES

CHILDREN, DIVORCE & STEPFAMILIES

CHILDREN & STRESS

RAISING RESILIENT KIDS

Community Educator Opportunity

Dear __________ :

The Alpha Centre is holding an open house for all School Psychologists and Guidance Counselors in the Anytown School District. The date of the open House is November 23, 1999, during National Education Week. This is an opportunity for us to network and learn of one another's services and needs.

Would you please send me a list of the names and addresses of the School Psychologist and Guidance Counselors who are employed by the District, so I can send them a personal invitation?

An announcement of the Open House is enclosed as well as one of our informational brochures and a newsletter. Please feel free to contact us about our counseling, consulting and psychoeducational services.

Thank you for your assistance. I will call you next week regarding the Open House.

Sincerely,

P.S. If you would like more brochures or newsletters, please give me a call.

FIGURE 6.4 Letter to Educators Announcing Open House

Dear ___________ :

I believe the following workshop can help Teachers improve their teaching techniques. On September 16, 1999, I am offering a two-session group for educators entitled:

Educators and the Myers-Briggs Type Indicator (MBTI): What Your Type Has to Say About Your Teaching Style and How to Improve Your Performance.

There will be a workshop for elementary and middle-school teachers, as well as one for high school teachers. Would you please bring these opportunities to the attention of your teachers in the Sunnyvale School District. I will facilitate the workshops and am a licensed marriage and family therapist with over twelve years experience. I am certified in the use of the Myers-Briggs and have found it to be a wonderful tool to help understand learning styles.

The workshops will meet for two hours on two consecutive Thursday evenings from 7:00 - 9:00 PM. Costs will be $50 plus $16 for test-taking and scoring. Groups meet at the Sunnyvale Community Center. Elementary and middle-school teachers meet on September 16 and 23; high school teachers on September 30 and October 7. Educator continuing education credits are also offered.

My program is also adaptable as an in-service training for your teachers, making it more convenient for them to attend.

Enclosed is an announcement, brochure, and informational newsletter.

If you wish have any questions, please contact me at (781) 322-3051. I will also call you within the next week.

Sincerely,

FIGURE 6.5 Letter to Educators Announcing Workshops

Dear __________ :

I am currently seeing a student of yours, David Smith. He and his parents entered counseling to deal with issues regarding David's classroom behavior. The enclosed release allows us to discuss his case freely.

I would like to arrange a meeting with you to review David's current situation and to gain a sense of his daily activities and movements.

David and his parents have shared their appreciation regarding your support of David during his transition to a new community and school. I believe that working together we can be helpful to everyone involved.

I am enclosing a brochure for your information and a complimentary newsletter, and will call you next week to arrange a mutually convenient appointment, and am looking forward to meeting with you.

Sincerely,

P.S. If you have any questions or concerns, please contact me immediately.

FIGURE 6.6 Cover Letter to Educator Accompanying Release Form

Referral Resource Information Sheet

When you do a new mailing, always include a Resource Directory Worksheet (see Figure 6.8) in order to build your community referral network. Have it available at your booth during conferences.

Communication needs to be two-way. Whenever you create a mailing, invite a response by including a mail-back card. You can also suggest to the recipients that they can telephone you if they have questions or comments.

Dear ___________ :

We want to make your work easier. As parents and professionals, we believe that educators, parent-teacher organizations, and the educational community are primary resources for supporting and enhancing the well-being of our community. We believe schools are an important component in meeting people's needs for community and life-meaning and are writing you because we believe our services can support you and the PTO in your important efforts. We know PTO's are an important component in meeting our town's needs for community and well-being.

The Alpha Centre for Counseling and Mediation seeks to serve the needs of the schools, parents and children of Malden, Medford, Melrose and surrounding communities by being available during a life crisis, and preventing problems through psychoeducation. We have many years of counseling experience, and provide services which enhance individuals, couples, children family and group relationships thereby improving the emotional and mental well-being of our communities. A brochure describing our services is enclosed along with an educational newsletter our clients and colleagues find helpful.

To help educate the community, we speak before civic groups, lead workshops, seminars and retreats on topics which may be helpful and of interest to your teachers and parent groups. Topics you may find interesting are printed on the side bar to the left. Additionally, we will work with you on topics related to you particular interests and needs.

We are sensitive to and respectful of diversity, multicultural and confidentiality issues. We are interested in meeting and discussing with you ways in which we might serve as resources to one another. We will call within the next week to arrange an interview date.

Sincerely,

FIGURE 6.7 Sample Introductory Letter to PTO

Date: ____________ New: ________ Revision: ________

Name: ______________________________________

School or Parent-Teacher Organization: ______________________

Address: ______________________________________

Telephone(s): ______________________________________

Fax: ____________________ E-mail Address: ______________

Web site: ______________________________________

Office Hours: ______________________________________

Relationship to School: ______________________________

Specialties: ______________________________________

Year Graduated: __________ College/University: ______________

Professional Memberships: ______________________________

____

Languages Spoken: ______________________________

What else is important that we know about you, your school, or your organization?

____

Thank you for completing this Resource Directory Form:

Mail to:

Alpha Centre
6 Pleasant Street, Suite 214
Malden, MA 02148

If you have any questions, please call (781)-322-3051.

Linda Lawless, MA, LMFT/LMHC/CCT; Jean Wright, D.Min, LMFT/L

Source: Adapted from L. Lawless, *Therapy Inc.* (New York: John Wiley, 1997). Reprinted with permission.

FIGURE 6.8 Educator and Education Community Resource Directory Worksheet

Telephone Script

Preparing. The educator or educational leader you are calling has received your letter and brochure in advance:

- Have a copy of the materials before you.
- Review your family-of-origin genogram as it relates to any relationships to the educational community and be comfortable with the relationships.
- Call when you are feeling refreshed and confident.
- Be prepared to not make contact on the first call; do not hesitate to call back.
- Be prepared to focus and take charge of the call since educators and educational leaders are busy professionals.
- Take a deep breath and place the call.

Connecting:

- You reach a receptionist or secretary. Identify yourself and your practice and ask to speak with Mr./Ms. "Smith" (educator/educational leader/educational resource). Share that you are responding to his or her request for information if the mail-back card has been returned. If not, say that you are calling to discuss your mailing with him or her. If you know a person in common, let the receptionist or secretary know who has referred or recommended Educator Smith to you. You will most likely receive a high priority. If he or she is not available, ask that your call be returned, leaving your telephone number with times you may be reached. If you do not receive a return call within a day or two, do not hesitate to call again. Remember that educators are busy professionals. Create a follow-up note to call again.
- You reach the educator. Have your script at hand and follow it. Keep your text to one page and remember that the call is about building a relationship. In your first paragraph, you begin building the relationship. Introduce yourself and your business; mention that you are a licensed mental health professional:

  This is ______, of ______. I'm a licensed ______ and have been located in [name of community] since ______. [If you know someone who knows the educator, mention the person's name and your relationship to him or her at this time. Let this person also know that you will be calling the educator. Share a positive bit of input, for example, "Barbara/Paul shared with me that you have a deep interest in supporting children/families where divorce is being experienced."]

(Continued)

Presentation. This comprises the second paragraph and contains your reason for calling.

> "Did you receive the letter and brochure I mailed on ______? Do you have questions, comments about it? "

Share why you want to network with educators (your particular specialties, which correlate with the educator's areas of expertise) and that you believe that you share mutual interests, which can benefit you both.

- Ask how long have they been teaching/involved with the PTO? How did they become interested in teaching, children of divorce? Be interested and keep your questions specific to the topic.
- Ask if they have worked with mental health professionals before. Mention common ground you feel is shared between the two professions (assisting and building healthy community). You may also base comments on your mission statement. Invite the educator's ideas about common ground (e.g., families of divorce) and include comments about your training and experience in the field. Share that you respect confidentiality issues. This will aid in building the bridges of trust and openness with them. For example, "Have you worked with mental health professionals before? If so, what has been your experience?"
- Ask if there are regular meetings of the educators to which you might be invited. If so, whom should you contact? Offer yourself as a speaker on a topic of interest to them. Can he or she be helpful or is there another contact? If so, who is that person?

Close. Your third paragraph brings closure to the telephone meeting. If all has gone well and you feel that there is a like-minded interest, invite the educator to lunch or ask for an appointment to meet and further discuss how you might assist one another. Make appropriate thank-yous and close with a "looking forward to meeting you in person" statement.

Affirming. Give yourself a pat on the back! You're on your way to building a niche market.

Completing. Follow up the telephone call with a note stating that you appreciate the time taken and that you look forward to the possibility of working together around your common interests. If you have scheduled a luncheon meeting and/or appointment to meet, mention it.

Developing a newsletter for the particular professional groups with which you network is another helpful way to gain name recognition and grow your practice. Depending on the time you have, it can be monthly or quarterly. Your feature article needs to focus on what will be informative and of interest to the reader.

To Do List

- Look in the Yellow Pages under Schools and select those that are compatible with your point of entry goals. (Public schools are usually listed under the town or city in which they are located.) Private schools will be in the Yellow Pages.
- Look in the Yellow Pages for your psychological association referral service and obtain names/addresses/telephone numbers of school psychologists in your area. Also, look under school psychologists and/or your state school psychologists association.
- Check educational web sites for your state and locality by [date].
- Check specialty schools and or special interest education focus groups for common ground by [date].
- Make list of educators/involved parents you already know, gather addresses, and telephone numbers by [date] to call them for possible referrals to other educators.
- List friends, family, and colleagues who may know educators and/or involved parents and the [date] you will call them.
- Prepare mailing to those on your point of entry list by [date].
- Develop brochure by [date].
- Write cover letters by [date].
- Develop and write enclosures by [date].
- Develop and write newsletter by [date].
- Mail packet by [date].
- Pick a calendar calling date.
- Review telephone script and practice aloud by [date].
- Integrate all dates with your Goals Plan by [date].
- Mail note by [date].

Telephone Script

Educators have very busy schedules and often are returning calls in the evening. If you choose to call and introduce yourself and/or respond to material you have received from an educator, keep the call focused, precise, and brief. Follow up with a note. The script on pages 189–190 is a guide for directing the conversation:

"To Do" List

A "To Do" list facilitates accountability and helps you focus your resources. A sample list is on page 191.

Summary

Use the information and resources in this chapter to build networks with the educational community. This information may also serve as a basis for seeking further information or research into the educational system.

Resources

Organizations and Websites

(Web sites often have links to state and local affiliates as well as links to numerous other related sites.)

Alliance for Parental Involvement in Education (ALLPIE)
P.O. Box 59
East Chatham, NY 12060-0059
(518) 392-6900
www.croton.com/allpie

American Association of Colleges for Teacher Education
One DuPont Circle, Suite 610
Washington, DC 20036-2412
(202) 293-2450

American Association of School Administrators
1801 North Moore Street
Arlington, VA 22209
(703) 528-0700
Fax: (703) 841-1543
www.aasa.org

American Association of University Professors (AAUP)
1012 Fourteenth Street NW, Suite 500
Washington, DC 20005-3465
(202) 737-5900
Fax: (202) 737-5526
www.aaup.org/

American Federation of Teachers
555 New Jersey Avenue NW
Washington, DC 20001
(202) 879-4400
www.aft.org

Association for School Counseling Professionals
801 North Fairfax Street, Suite 310
Alexandria, VA 22314
(703) 683-2722
Fax: (703) 683-1619
www.schoolcounselor.org/

Clearinghouse on Disabilities and Gifted Education (ERIC)
www.cec.sped.org/ericec.htm

Colorado Parent Information and Resource Center
Center for Human Investment Policy
1445 Market Street, Suite 350
Denver, CO 80202
(303) 820-5632
Fax: (303) 820-5656
www.cpirc.org/

Education Commission of the States (ECS)
707 17th Street, Suite 2700
Denver, CO 80202-3427
(303) 229-3600
Fax: (303) 296-8332
www.ecs.org

Education News and Resources (Free e-mail newsletter)
2211 Spruce Street
Port Townsend, WA 98368
(360) 385-4387
www.edbriefs.com/

Hand-in-Hand: Parents, Schools, Communities United for Kids
1001 Connecticut Avenue NW, Suite 310
Washington, DC 20036
(202) 822-8405
Fax: (202) 872-4050

The Institute for Educational Leadership, Inc.
1001 Connecticut Avenue NW, Suite 310
Washington, DC 20036
(202) 822-8405
Fax: (202) 872-4050

National Association for the Education of Young Children (NAEYC)
1509 16th Street NW
Washington, DC 20036
(800) 424-2460
Fax: (202) 328-1846
www.naeyc.org/

National Association of Elementary School Principals
1615 Duke Street
Alexandria, VA 22314
(800) 38-NAESP
Fax: (800) 39-NAESP
www.naesp.org/

National Association of Secondary School Principals
1904 Association Drive
Reston, VA 20191
(703) 860-0200
Fax: (703) 476-5432
www.nassp.org/

National Association for Family Child Care
206 Sixth Avenue, Suite 900
Des Moines, IA 50309
(800) 359-3817
www.nafcc.org.

National Association for Gifted Children
1707 L Street NW, Suite 550
Washington, DC 20036
(202) 785-4268
www.nagc.org/

National Coalition for Parent Involvement in Education (NCPIE)
1201 16th Street NW, Box 39
Washington, DC 20036
(202) 822-8405
Fax: (202) 872-4050
www.ncpie.org/

National Council for Accreditation of Teacher Education (NCATE)
2010 Massachusetts Avenue NW, Suite 500
Washington, DC 20036-1023
(202) 466-7496

National Education Association
1201 16th Street NW
Washington, DC 20036
(202) 833-4000
www.nea.org/

National Parent-Teachers Association (PTA)
330 N. Wabash Avenue, Suite 2100
Chicago, IL 60611
(312) 670-6782
www.pta.org

National School Boards Association
1680 Duke Street
Alexandria, VA 22314
(703) 838-6722
Fax: (703) 683-7590
www.nsba.org

J. Brien O'Callaghan, Ph.D., LMFT
54 Plum Trees Road
Bethel, CT 060801
(203) 790-4498
e-mail: drbrien@jbocallaghan.com
web site: http://www.jbocallahgan.com

U.S. Department of Education
400 Maryland Avenue SW
Washington, DC 20202-0498
(800) USA-LEARN
www.ed.gov/

The U.S. Department of Health and Human Services
200 Independence Avenue SW
Washington, DC 20201
(877) 696-6775
www.os.dhhs.gov/

National Parent Information Network
www.npin.org

ERIC Clearinghouse on Elementary and Early Childhood Education
University of Illinois
Children's Research Center
51 Gerty Drive
Champaign, IL 61820-7469
(217) 333-1386

Center for Applied Research in Education
110 Brookhill Drive
West Nyack, NY 10995-9901
www.prenhall.com

Children's Advocacy Organizations

Children's Defense Fund—www.childrensdefense.org

Stand for Children—www.stand.org

National Committee to Prevent Child Abuse—www.childabuse.org

Coalition to Stop Gun Violence—www.gunfree.org

Violence Policy Center—www.vpc.org

Center for Media Education—www.cme.org

National Clearinghouse on Child Abuse/Neglect—www.hai-net.com/nccan/nccan.htm

Advocates for Youth—www.advocatesforyouth.org

KIDS FIRST!—www.cqcm.org/kidsfirst. Rates children's media.

For Parents of Children with Chronic Illness and/or Disabilities

Asthma and Allergy Foundation of America
1125 15th Street NW, Suite 502
Washington, DC 20005
(800) 7-ASTHMA

Allergy and Asthma Network/Mothers of Asthmatics
3554 Chain Bridge Road, Suite 200
Fairfax, VA 22030-2709
(800) 878-4403
www.podi.com/health/aanma

CHADD (Children and Adults with Attention Deficit Disorders)
8181 Professional Place, Suite 201
Landover, MD 20785
(800) 233-4050
Fax: (301) 306-7090
www.chadd.org/

The Council for Exceptional Children
1920 Association Drive
Reston, VA 20191-1589
(888) CEC-SPED
www.cec.sped.org/

International Dyslexia Association
8600 LaSalle Road
Chester Building, Suite 382
Baltimore, MD 21286-2044
(410) 296-0232
www.interdys.org/

KidsPeace: The National Center for Kids Overcoming Crisis
1650 Broadway
Bethlehem, PA 18015-3998
(800) 25-PEACE
www.kidspeace.org

Resource for parents of deaf children—www.cuedspeech.com

For Assistance with Infants and Young Children who are developmentally disabled:

The Let's Play! Project at the University of Buffalo, New York, Center for Assistive Technology—http://cosmos.ot.buffalo.edu/letsplay/ call: Sue Mistrett at (716) 829-3141.

National Information Center for Children and Youth with Disabilities
P.O. Box 1492
Washington, DC 20013-1492
(800) 695-0285

Parents of Kids with Infectious Diseases (PKIDS)
P.O. Box 5666
Vancouver, WA 98668
(360) 695-0293
Fax: (360) 695-6941
www. pkids.org/pkids.htm

Mental Health

American Academy of Child and Adolescent Psychiatry
3615 Wisconsin Avenue NW
Washington, DC 20016
(800) 333-7636

Center for Mental Health Services
Knowledge Exchange Network
P.O. Box 42490
Washington, DC 20015
(800) 789-2647

Family Resource Coalition
200 South Michigan Avenue, 16th Floor
Chicago, IL 60604
(312) 341-0900

Federation of Families for Children's Mental Health
1021 Prince Street
Alexandria, VA 22314
(703) 684-7710

National Mental Health Association: Children's Mental Health
1021 Prince Street
Alexandria, VA 22314
(800) 969-6642
www.nmha.org/

Occupational Information (Teachers)

Bureau of Labor Statistics, Occupational Employment Statistics: http://stats.bls.gov/oes/oes_data.htm
Bureau of Labor Statistics, Occupational Outlook Handbook: http://stats.bls.gov/ocohome.htm
Department of Education, National Center for Education Statistics: http://nces.ed.gov/indihome.asp

Financial Aid

The Financial Aid Information page—www.finaid.org
Collegenet—www.collegenet.com

Homework

Study Web—www.studyweb.com

B.J. Pinchbeck's Homework Helper—www.bjpinchbeck.com

Homeschooling

Homeschool Helper—www.mathgoodies.com/homeschool

Home Schooling Made Easy!—http://core-curriculum.com

The Education Station—www.edstation.com

Home Schooling Daily: www.infinet.com/~baugust/theme.html

Learning in the Real World—www.realworld.org

Art Projects for Children—www.kinderart.com

Catalogs

At-Risk Resources
135 Dupont Street
P.O. Box 760
Plainview, NY 11803-1760
(800) 999-6884
www.at-risk.com

Childswork/ChildsPlay
P.O. Box 1604
Secaucus, NJ 07096-1604
(800) 962-1141
Fax: (201) 583-3644

KIDSRIGHTS
10100 Park Cedar Drive
Charlotte, NC 28210
(800) 892-KIDS

National Observances

National High School Education Month—November; National Association of Secondary School Principals (see listing under Organizations and web sites)

National Parents' Day—July 27; Parents' Day Foundation (703) 790-8700

Library Card Sign Up Month—September; American Library Association (312) 280-5041

International Literacy Day—September; National Institute for Literacy (202) 632-1500

America Goes Back to School Week—U.S. Department of Education (see listing under Organizations and web sites)

Child Health Month—October, American Academy of Pediatrics (847) 228-5005

Computer Learning Month—October, Computer Learning Foundation (415) 327-3347

National Fire Prevention Week—October 5–11, National Fire Protection Association (617) 984-7270

Child Health Day—October 6, American Health Foundation (212) 953-1900

National School Celebration—October 10, Celebration USA (714) 283-1892

National School Bus Safety Week—October 19–25, National School Transportation Association (703) 644-0700

National Chemistry Week—November 2–8, American Chemical Society (800) 227-5558, ext. 6097

National Geography Awareness Week—November 16–22, National Geographic Society (800) 368-2728

American Education Week—November 16–22, National Education Association (NEA) (202) 822-7200

National Take Our Parents to School Week—November 16–22, Hand in Hand/Institute for Educational Leadership (202) 822-8405, ext. 25

National Children's Book Week, Children's Book Council (212) 966-1990

National Community Education Day—November, National Community Education Association (703) 359-8973

National Education Support Personnel Day—November, National Education Association (NEA) (202) 822-7200

National Drunk and Drugged Driving Prevention Month—December, U.S. Department of Transportation (202) 366-2020

World AIDS Day—December 1, American Association for World Health (202) 466-5883

To order a calendar that indicates special observances:

Health Observances and Recognition Day Calendar—contact: Society for Healthcare Strategy and Market Development (800) 242-2626.

Chase's Calendar of Events—The Day-to-Day Directory to Special Days, Weeks, and Months (312) 540-4500.

Recommended Reading

Bell, R. (Ed.). (1980). *Changing bodies, changing lives: A book for teens on sex and relationships.* New York: Random House.

Berne, P., & Savary, L. (1981). *Building self-esteem in children.* New York: Continuum Press.

Bickman, L., & Rog, D.J. (Eds.). (1995). *Children's mental health services: Research, policy, and evaluation, "School-based mental health services for children,"* pp. 117–144. Thousand Oaks, CA: Sage.

Blanch, G. (1987). *The subtle seductions: How to be a "good enough" parent.* Northvale, NJ: Jason Aronson.

Blum, D.J. (1988). *The school counselor's book of lists.* West Nyack, NY: Center for Applied Research in Education.

Bode, J. (1998). *Food fight: A guide to eating disorders for preteens and their parents.* New York: Aladdin Paperbacks.

Brameld, T.B.H. (1971). *Patterns of educational philosophy: Divergence and convergence in culturological perspective.* New York: Holt, Rinehart and Winston.

Brenner, A. (1985). *Helping children cope with stress.* Lexington, MA: Lexington Books.

Briesmeister, J.M., & Schaefer, C.E. (Eds.). (1998). *Handbook of parent training: Parents as co-therapists for children's behavior problems* (2nd ed.). New York: Wiley.

Briggs, D. (1970). *Your child's self-esteem: The key to life.* New York: Doubleday.

Canfield, J., & Well, H. (1976). *100 ways to enhance self-concept in the classroom.* Englewood Cliffs, NJ: Prentice Hall.

Caplan, G. (1964). *Principles of preventive psychiatry.* New York: Basic Books.

Caron, A.F. (1994). *Strong mothers, strong sons: Raising adolescent boys in the '90s.* New York: Henry Holt.

Carter, E.A., & McGoldrick, M.. (Eds.). (1980). *The family life cycle: A framework for family therapy.* New York: Gardner Press.

Cloud, H., & Townsend, J. (1988). *Boundaries with kids.* Grand Rapids, MI: Zondervan.

Coles, R. (1986). *The moral life of children: How children struggle with questions of moral choice in the United States and elsewhere.* Boston, MA: Houghton Mifflin.

Coopersmith, S. (1967). *The antecedents of self-esteem.* San Francisco: Freeman.

Dalsimer, K. (1986). *Female adolescence: Psychoanalytic reflections on literature.* New Haven, CT: Yale University Press.

Duska, R., & Whelan, M. (1975). *Moral development: A guide to Piaget and Kohlberg.* New York: Paulist Press.

Edwards, Y., & Edwards, M. (1989). *Becoming a powerful parent.* Auckland: Hodder & Stoughton.

Elium, D., & Elium, J. (1992). *Raising a son: Parents and the making of a healthy man.* Berkeley, CA: Celestial Arts.

Erickson, E.H. (1963). *Childhood and society* (2nd ed.). New York: Norton.

Erickson, E.H. (Ed.). (1965). *The challenge of youth.* Garden City, NY: Anchor Books.

Erickson E.H. (1980). *Identity and the life cycle.* New York: Norton.

Faber, A., & Mazlish, E. (1982). *How to talk so kids will listen, how to listen so kids will talk.* New York: Avon Books.

Feldman, J.R. (1997). *Ready-to-use self-esteem activities for young children.* West Nyack, NY: Center for Applied Research in Education.

Finch, A.J., Jr., Nelson, W.M., III, & Ott, E.S. (1993). *Cognitive-behavioral procedures with children and adolescents: A practical guide.* Boston: Allyn & Bacon.

Freire, P. (1994). *Pedagogy of the oppressed.* New York: Continuum.

Frick, W.B. (1971). *Humanistic psychology: Interviews with Maslow, Murphy, and Rogers.* Columbus, OH: Merrill.

Gilligan, C. (1982). *In a different voice: Psychological theory and women's development.* Cambridge, MA: Harvard University Press.

Gilligan, C., Lyons, N.P., & Hanmer, T.J. (1989). *Making connections: The relational worlds of adolescent girls at Emma Willard School.* Troy, NY: Emma Willard School.

Ginott, H. (19720. *Between teachers and children.* New York: Macmillan.

Goetz, P.W. (Ed.). (1995). Higher education (pp. 1–11); History of education (pp. 11–100); Special education (pp. 111–114); Systems of education (pp. 115–132). In *Encyclopedia Britannica* (15th ed., Vol. 18). Chicago: University of Chicago.

Goleman, D. (1995). *Emotional intelligence: Why it can matter more than IQ.* New York: Bantam Books.

Grunebaum, H. (Ed.). (1970). *The practice of community mental health.* Boston: Little, Brown.

Guntrip, H. (1973). *Psychoanalytic theory, therapy, and the self: A basic guide to the human personality in Freud, Erikson, Klein, Sullivan, Fairbairn, Hartmann, Jacobson, and Winnicott.* New York: Basic Books.

Haley, J. (1980). *Leaving home: The therapy of disturbed young people.* New York: McGraw-Hill.

Harris, M. (1988). *Women and teaching: Themes for a spirituality of pedagogy.* New York: Paulist Press.

Hauser, S.T. (with Powers, S.I., and Noam, G.G.). (1991). *Adolescents and their families: Paths of ego development.* New York: Free Press.

Hart, L. (1987). *The winning family.* New York: Mead.

Imber-Black, E. (1998). *The secret life of families: Truth-telling, privacy, and reconciliation in a tell-all society.* New York: Bantam Books.

Jordan, J.V., Kaplan, A.G., Miller, J.B., Stiver, I.P., & Surrey, J.L. (1991). *Women's growth in connection: Writings from the Stone Center.* New York: Guilford Press.

Joseph, J. (1994). *The resilient child.* New York: Plenum Press.

Kaplan, L. (1986). *Working with multiproblem families.* Lexington, MA: Lexington Books.

Kaplan, L., & Girard, J.L. (1994). *Strengthening high-risk families: A handbook for practitioners.* New York: Lexington Books.

Kegan, R. (1982). *The evolving self: Problem and process in human development.* Cambridge, MA: Harvard University Press.

Kegan, R. (1994). *In over our heads: The mental demands of modern life.* Cambridge, MA: Harvard University Press.

Kiersey, D., & Bates, M. (1984). *Please understand me: Character and temperament types.* Del Mar, CA: Prometheus Nemesis.

Kelly, M. (1998). *The mother's almanac goes to school: Your child from six to twelve.* New York: Doubleday.

Lawless, L.L. (1997). *Therapy, Inc. A hands-on guide to developing, positioning, and marketing your mental health practice in the 90s.* New York: Wiley.

Lawrence, G.D. (1995). *Descriptions of the sixteen types.* Gainesville, FL: Center for Applications of Psychological Type.

Lickona, T. (1991). *Educating for character: How our schools can teach respect and responsibility.* New York: Bantam Books.

March, J.S. (Ed.). (1995). *Anxiety disorders in children and adolescents.* New York: Guilford Press.

Melton, G.B., & Barry, F.D. (Eds.). (1994). *Protecting children from abuse and neglect.* New York: Guilford Press.

Mungazi, D.A. (1998). *The evolution of educational theory in the United States.* Westport, CT: Praeger.

Myers, I.B., & McCaulley, M.H. (1985). *Manual: A guide to the development and use of the Myers-Briggs type indicator.* Palo Alto, CA: Consulting Psychology Press.

O'Callaghan, J.B. (1993). *School-based collaboration with families: Constructing family-school-agency partnerships that work.* New York: Jossey-Bass.

Osherson, S. (1995). *The passions of fatherhood.* New York: Fawcett Columbine.

Pipher, M. (1995). *Reviving Ophelia: Saving the selves of adolescent girls.* New York: Ballantine Books.

Pollack, W. (1998). *Real boys: Rescuing our sons from the myths of boyhood.* New York: Random House.

Ponton, L.E. (1997). *The romance of risk: Why teenagers do the things they do.* New York: Basic Books.

Rodriguez, C. (1998, November 27). Even in middle school, girls are thinking thin. *Boston Globe,* pp. B1, B9.

Rubin, T.I. (1990). *Child potential: Fulfilling your child's intellectual, emotional, and creative promise.* New York: Continuum.

Rutter, M., & Rutter, M. (1993). *Developing minds: Challenge and continuity across the life span.* New York: Basic Books.

Sarrel, L.J., & Sarrel, P.M. (1979). *Sexual unfolding: Sexual development and sex therapies in late adolescence.* Boston: Little, Brown.

Satir, V. (1972). *Peoplemaking.* Palo Alto, CA: Science and Behavior Books.

Schulman, M., & Mekler, E. (1985). *Bringing Up a moral child: A new approach for teaching your child to be kind, just, and responsible.* Reading, MA: Addison-Wesley.

Sears, M., & Sears, W.M. (1995). *The discipline book: Everything you need to know to have a better-behaved child—from birth to age ten.* Boston: Little, Brown.

Shore, K. (1994). *The parents' public school handbook: How to make the most of your child's education from kindergarten through middle school.* New York: Fireside.

Stacey, J., Bereaud, S., & Daniels, J. (1978). *And Jill came tumbling after: Sexism in American education.* New York: Dell.

Stevenson, L. (1987). *Seven theories of human nature: Christianity, Freud, Lorenz, Marx, Sartre, Skinner, and Plato* (2nd ed.). Oxford, England: Oxford University Press.

Stewart, A.J., Copeland, A.P., Chester, N.L., Malley, J.E., & Barenbaum, N.B. (1997). *Separating together: How divorce transforms families.* New York: Guilford Press.

Strain, J.P. (1971). *Modern philosophies of education.* New York: Random House.

Textor, M.R. (1983). *Helping families with special problems.* New York: Jason Aronson.

Toman, W. (1993). *Family therapy and sibling position*. Northvale, NJ: Jason Aronson.

U.S. Department of Education, National Center for Education Statistics, *Digest of Education Statistics*. http://nces.ed.gov/indihome.asp

Visher, E.B., & Visher, J.S. (1982). *How to win as a step-family*. New York: Brunner/Mazel.

Wood, B.L. (1992). *Raising healthy children in an alcoholic home*. New York: Crossroad.

7

Strategic Marketing to Managed Care Organizations

If you begin to work with MCOs and perform badly, the negative record in your provider profile may jeopardize future referrals.

At first glance, approaching managed care can appear quite daunting, if not overwhelming. Although managed care is a large and complex specialized marketplace, it can be lucrative. Whether you feel prepared for or comfortable spending your time and energy on this market is a different issue. Before taking the first step, complete the self-assessment on page 204. Record your readiness to pursue managed care organizations in each of the following areas.

Managed care is a healthcare management *system*, mental healthcare being only one piece of that system. Each system member has its own values and needs. The broad-brush definition of managed care is "any system that contains utilization management, case management, provider selection, and cost containment" (Lawless, 1997). Members of a mental health managed-care system include:

- The mental health professional.
- The client or consumer.
- The employer or association that provides the healthcare plan.
- The managed care organization.
- National and regional laws, legislation, and regulatory functions.

As a provider, you can reach out to the potential client, the employer or association or the managed-care organization (MCO) itself. However, this niche market has its own language. If you are new to this arena, you need to get a copy of a glossary and keep it handy as you speak to people in this system (see Resources for glossary sources).

Managed care grew out of the biomedicalization of mental health and the use of the *Diagnostic and Statistical Manual of Mental Disorders*

Score on a scale from 1–5, 1 = Never or No; 5 = Always or Yes; 2,3,4, being degrees in between.

____ I return telephone calls promptly.
____ I am a team player.
____ I have coverage for my practice when I am not available (e.g., vacation, emergencies, or business travel).
____ My emergency backups have access to my records when I am away.
____ I have psychopharm consultants I can refer to.
____ I manage my tasks well and can get reports in on time.
____ I keep thorough clinical records.
____ I do my billing promptly and accurately.
____ I can write goal-oriented treatment plans.
____ I track my clients' progress with clear and measurable progress steps.
____ I can verbally conceptualize a case and discuss it with colleagues.
____ I use informed consent and information release forms regularly.
____ I carry maximum malpractice insurance.
____ I manage my cases to include community and other self-help resources in the overall treatment plan.
____ I understand and can use the *DSM-IV*.
____ I have short-term treatment skills.
____ I have formal training in my specialty areas.
____ My office is client friendly.
____ I have a practice management system that tracks treatment authorizations and billings.
____ I keep accurate and timely financial records.
____ I have at least three years of post-master's experience.
____ I can clearly and concisely describe my treatment philosophy.

____ Total Score

Scoring: If you scored less than 110, you are not ready to work with managed care. We highly recommend getting these aspects of your practice in order before taking on this niche market. Be cautious and carefully plan your decision to work with managed care companies, because if you begin to work with MCOs and perform badly, the negative record in your provider profile may jeopardize future referrals. Also, if you have a philosophical disagreement about the values, goals, and strategies of MCOs (e.g., cost-effective, performance-related treatment), then you need to rethink the relationship, and ask yourself if you can work within their structure.

(*DSM-IV*; American Psychiatric Association, 1994). "The *DSM* provides a means to equate dollar amounts to mental illness in much the same way as equating the cost of a broken leg to average medical procedures" (Lawless, 1997).

Over the past 17 years, managed care organizations (MCOs) have become an industry, that has changed the face of mental healthcare delivery. New laws and legislation have played a significant role in this change and will continue to alter the system. Some of the changes the managed-care movement has created are a reduction in fees and clientele as well as a greater accountability for professionals, a reduction in the use of mental health insurance usage, and less psychiatric hospitalization time. The MCO clinical trend has been toward short-term, strategic clinical treatment that stresses effective practice management with positive cash flow, quick response time, timely treatment planning, and subsequent authorization or denial. Some practitioners can move into this arena and survive, sometimes flourish. Others have great difficulty with this system and need to look for other niche markets. Mergers have resulted in a few big players that manage the majority of participants in this industry.

The MCO clinical trend has been toward a short-term, strategic clinical treatment model that stresses effective practice management.

The level of sophistication of the managed care industry varies from state to state and within regions in each state. In Massachusetts, there are two major Stage 4 areas, with the outlying areas being more typical of Stage 3. The following stages of development will help you identify where your region stands:

Stage 1. Unstructured care is the norm; there is little managed care or hospital consolidation. Individual providers use fee-for-service, indemnity plans, and some managed care.

Stage 2. A loose framework begins to form in which most managed care consists of discounted fee-for-service care. Hospital consolidation begins, insurers begin to acquire or partner with providers, provider groups form, and an oversupply of mental health beds supports deep price discounts. The individual provider is often included in provider panels.

Stage 3. Consolidation occurs with heavy managed-care penetration into regional and government programs and also private plans. Managed care dominates as a payment source. Some capitation is used, hospital mergers and acquisitions take place, and some plans begin dropping providers. As managed care consolidates itself, providers and insurers begin to align. The individual provider finds it more difficult to get a position on panels.

Stage 4. Managed-care competition takes shape. Employer coalitions buy healthcare contracts and managed-care payment dominates the marketplace rather than fee-for-service arrangements. A few large healthcare players dominate the region. Providers and insurers are strongly aligned. Networks develop a full continuum of subacute care. Providers and insurers organize to serve covered lives. More than 50 percent of people insured use an HMO. The individual provider has difficulty getting on panels (Lawless, 1997).

Phases of Managed Care

Individual MCOs go through phases of development just as people do. If you are targeting or are currently working with an MCO, ask yourself which of the following developmental levels it has reached:

First Generation. Reduces costs by restricting access to services through rigid utilization reviews, provides limited benefits, and requires large copayments. It is easiest to market to this marketplace.

Second Generation. Begins the creation of provider networks, selective contracting, increased treatment planning, and is less rigid in utilization reviews.

Third Generation. Manages the care of patients by emphasizing treatment planning and more active client management during treatment. It allows the use of the least restrictive treatment settings that are clinically appropriate.

Fourth Generation. Manages by outcomes. Greater provider autonomy achieves successful outcomes by creating a self-correcting treatment system. This marketplace is much more complex and difficult to enter.

The Diversity of MCOs

There are many types of MCO structures, each covering a specific population with a varied benefit plan. Here are the major types of MCO entities:

- *Commercial Carriers.* Payments are made to qualified providers based on a schedule of benefits for specified services. These carriers often do not have a provider panel.
- *Fee-for-Service.* A benefit package with no network direction consisting of a high degree of choice and flexibility such as Blue Cross/Blue Shield. These MCOs often have provider panels and may also pay out-of-panel providers, who are paid at a lower rate than in-panel providers.
- *Self-Insured Welfare Plan.* Benefits are provided directly by an employer or through an employee union or retirement plan such as the Retail Clerks Union Plan.
- *Health Maintenance Organization (HMO).* These MCOs are often called a "staff model" since providers are usually employees of the HMO. Referrals to outside providers are made only when no in-house provider can cover the consumer's need. Members pay monthly premiums and often also have copayments, which they pay at the time of service. Two examples are Kaiser Permanente and the Harvard/Vanguard Community Health Plan.

These MCOs are often called a "staff model" since providers are usually employees of the HMO.

- *Preferred Provider Organization (PPO).* This is a group of providers who have contractually agreed to provide services for a standard fee set by, or negotiated with, the MCO. Many MCOs create their own PPO. Usually subscribers have a deductible, pay an annual fee, and have some form of copay for services received. An example is United Behavioral HealthCare.
- *Employee Assistance Program (EAP).* This is an in-house or external system that assesses employees' needs and recommends treatment options. Some EAPs have in-house services, but many refer to providers outside their system. The referral providers usually are noncontractual. The client can have some kind of mental health insurance that picks up treatment when the EAP benefit is exceeded. If you are an EAP provider, you sometimes cannot then be the provider who works with the subsequent insurance carrier.
- *Medical Savings Account (MSA).* Employees have pretaxable funds automatically deducted from their paycheck. They can use this money for any qualified provider.
- *Federal Employee Health Benefits (FEHB)—Civilian Health and Medical Program of the Uniformed Services (CHAMPUS); Medicare;*

Medicaid. These government programs have their own list of acceptable participating providers. These systems are currently in the process of converting to an MCO model.

- *Workers' Compensation.* These are benefits for employees who suffer injury or disability as a result of job-related accidents or occupational diseases. For a complete breakdown on workers' compensation laws for your state, write to the U.S. Chamber of Commerce, Publications Dept., 1615 H Street NW, Washington, DC 20062 or telephone (202) 659-6000.

The Marketplace

Current Status

Entry into preferred provider lists is increasingly difficult but not impossible.

Managed care has forced the psychotherapy profession to identify how it facilitates healing or creates change. Some mental health professionals are concerned that the art of psychotherapy will be replaced by the industry of managed care. The market has been engulfing smaller entities and forming large megastructures. Entry onto preferred provider lists is increasingly difficult but not impossible. Fees are still on the low side and will probably continue to decrease. Risk is being transferred to the provider. Given all these disadvantages, why would anyone want to work in this marketplace? The answer is referrals. If you want to see who the major players are and what they are paying providers, check out an Internet site that lists reimbursement fees by CPT code—Mental Health Associates at http://mentalhealth-madison.com/Documents/Latest.htm. When you see the figures, you may skip to the next chapter.

The Future of MCOs

MCOs are competing to cover the majority of clients for mental health services. The larger the number of members covered, the more control they have over the marketplace. The following developments are predicted for the future, and some are already evolving into a reality:

- An integration of employee assistance programs, managed behavioral products, and workers' compensation.
- Medicare moving to a managed-care model.

- An integrated health data system for outcomes measures and provider performance ratings.
- Standardization of treatment methods often called practice standards.
- More government regulation on the practices of all levels of managed care.
- Increased use of outpatient group therapy.
- Early detection and treatment primarily made by the primary care physician (PCP).
- Treating the mind and body together.
- Increasing demand by the growing elderly population.
- Greater emphasis on wellness and prevention.

As the market matures, MCOs likely will offer multiproduct frameworks for different market segments:

- *Premium Product—Fee-for-Service.* This product is for highly paid employees who want to have maximum flexibility and choice. Employees and owners will have a pool of providers who have been identified by specialty services. There may or may not be a contractual agreement for reduced fees with the provider based on volume and availability.
- *Midrange Products—Preferred Provider Organization PPO.* This will be a traditional PPO as described earlier.
- *Exclusive Provider Organization (EPO) or Health Maintenance Organization (HMO) with a Point-of-Service Option.* This market segment will be made up of members willing to work with a gatekeeper and will retain the option of out-of-system benefits.
- *High-Volume Product—Basic Health Maintenance Organization.* This will be a pure HMO with the priority placed on cost savings rather than choice.

Needs of Managed-Care Organizations

In a few words, MCOs want "focused symptom reduction" (Browning 1994). They are looking for problem specific, well-defined goals, and treatment plans that can be tracked to reach those goals. They don't want long process-oriented descriptions of client needs, difficulty dealing with you, long-term care, hospitalizations, client complaints, and therapists who do not return calls promptly or get their paperwork in on time. Generally, they prefer group practices or individual practices located in an office setting, not in the home of the practitioner.

A direct inquiry is the best way to identify the MCO's needs.

A direct inquiry is the best way to identify the MCO's needs. Call the provider support person and ask this simple question, "What do I need to do to be sent more referrals?" If you want them to remember you, send progress reports and closing summaries when you are working with their client. Let them know about the workshops you attend and new services you are adding to your practice; develop a relationship with them. When you make a mistake, be sure to let them know before anyone else does and offer a way to correct the problem.

Differing MCO System Perspectives

Each member of the MCO system has an individual need system and his or her own perspective of the marketplace. We interviewed several members including a member of a group practice, an MCO employee, an MCO consultant, an alternative MCO system member, and a private practitioner. The responses to the following four questions were diverse:

1. How does managed care currently affect the practice of mental healthcare?
2. What do you foresee as the future of managed care?
3. What advice do you have for mental health professionals regarding MC?
4. What skills and strategies are needed for mental health professionals to work successfully with MCs?

All the interviewees shared insightful and helpful information (Ginter, Kelly, & Lawless, 1998). Overall, the private and group practitioners believed managed care was affecting the quality of care for clients and making it more difficult to practice. The MCO employee believed managed care had helped the profession by demanding accountability for treatment outcomes and using financial responsibility to provide services. The MCO consultant advised professionals to gain business skills and fulfill the requirements of MCOs, and the alternative MCO system member believed MCOs would extinguish the private practitioner and quality mental healthcare. Since there is no consensus in these perspectives, you must understand the position of any MCO individual or group, before deciding whether you want to work with them.

Analyzing Your Needs

Should You Join a Group?

Some MCOs will only contract with an integrated delivery system (IDS). That means they want one-stop shopping. They want to make one phone call and refer a client to a system that can meet most needs (i.e., specialty coverage, psychopharm, outcomes reporting, financial management, case management, relationships with hospitals, and primary care physicians). If you work well in a group practice, this may be the best solution for you since IDSs have been identified as the system of choice of MCOs in the future. There is a long start-up curve in creating an IDS in today's market; first look for an established one you can join. If you are in a first- or second-generation MCO region, your area may be ready for this kind of business start-up. There are many good managed-care consultants who can help you set up your group. Resources for consultants include *Psychotherapy Finances*, NASW, APA, and *Open Minds* (see Resources section for contact information).

If you want to continue in independent practice, then you will need to seek out MCOs who continue to contract with individual practitioners. As of this writing, there are still many out there. If you scored 110 on the self-assessment at the beginning of this chapter, you are ready to take on MCOs. If you are already working in this marketplace, you may want to increase your referrals. Try to keep a wide base of referrals and avoid basing your practice on a single source. The marketplace is fickle and you may find yourself one day with no referrals.

If you want to continue in independent practice, then you will need to seek out MCOs who continue to contract with individual practitioners.

Niche Experience

If you have had some experience working with MCOs, ask yourself which collaborations were the most enjoyable or at least trouble free. These are the companies where you want to expand your participation. The first question to ask is:

What makes you special? Why would a utilization manager or caseworker send a client to you? The primary reason should be because you serve the needs of the potential client. Other answers could be:

- There are others in your practice group covering a wide range of specialties and needs.
- Your paperwork for the MCO is on time and accurate.
- You have a reputation as a high-quality provider.
- You have a personal relationship with the referral sources.
- You are the only one in a geographic area.
- You understand and agree with their treatment philosophy.
- You have evening and weekend hours open.
- You have crisis response capability.
- You provide excellent treatment planning and discharge plans.
- You provide effective brief treatment.
- Your specialty is validated with formal documentation of training and experience.
- You refer for medication when indicated.
- You require client homework and bibliotherapy, and use community resources.
- Your documentation is consistent and problem oriented.
- You use pre- and postassessments for outcomes measures.
- You offer a customer satisfaction survey.
- You submit claims electronically.

Engaging the Marketplace

The first step is to think about the big picture and ask yourself which member of this system you feel the most comfortable working with. Would you prefer working with a local or national MCO? Would a small EAP in your community be a better match? Once you have narrowed the field, you can begin your search of MCOs.

Finding the Names of Appropriate MCOs

An MCO who wants to provide services in your state must register with them. You can request this list from your state insurance Commissioner.

Every state has an insurance commission. An MCO who wants to provide services in your state must register with them. You can request this list from your state insurance commissioner. You can find a list of state insurance regulators at the National Association of Insurance Commissioners web site—www.naic.org. There are also companies that sell names of MCOs. Contact your national professional association for a list of resources and look in the advertising section of professional publications. A resource we have used is the Professional Health Plan whose telephone number is (510) 601-8033. Also, you can subscribe to one of these managed-care periodicals and watch for announcements of open panels:

Psychotherapy Finances (407) 624-1155
Open Minds (717) 334-1329
Practice Management Monthly (800) 578-5013
Managed Care Strategies (800) 869-8450.

Making a Match

Here are some issues to consider when deciding to work with any MCO:

- Who carries the liability if the MCO makes a mistake? It should not be you.
- What kind of access do they have to your records?
- Do they have gag rules?
- How timely do they pay?
- What kind of process do they have for treatment authorization and reauthorization?
- Do they have a member directory?
- Where do referrals come from? Look for MCOs that proactively triage with a method for referring clients based on the client's needs and the therapist's skills.
- How much do they pay?

Some companies make working with them simple and straightforward, and others make it nearly impossible to maintain any kind of clarity about payment response and authorization. The answer about who you want to work with seems simple.

Marketing Plan

The first step in developing your MCO marketing plan is to put together a practice profile. This profile creates a word picture of you and your practice. Most of this information will be asked on the provider application. If it is not asked, include it in a cover letter with your application:

- What kinds of services you offer.
- Your availability for new clients (i.e., can make a first appointment within 24 hours).
- Hours of service.
- How "community friendly" your office is (e.g., wheelchair access, public transportation, well-lighted parking).
- How you respond to and manage emergencies and callbacks.
- The outcome results you can show a potential MCO panel.
- Your specialties and how you can verify training.
- The continuing education classes you took in the past three years.
- Academic credentials and any special training you have received.
- Number of years in practice.
- A practice assessment that lists client outcomes (i.e., diagnosis, number of sessions and cost per case).
- Your commitment to short-term strategic treatment. If you have done any outcome studies on your clients, you can include a practice summary with your letter.
- If you do any of your own testing, include what kind.
- If you have a practice brochure or newsletter, include a copy.
- Other MCOs you already work with. Do not include more than three.
- Second languages spoken.
- The reasons they would want to include you in their panel.
- The members of the practice and their specialties.

- How you assure quality. This could be an outcomes measurement system or a quality management process. The emphasis is how identified problems are used to correct or resolve problems after they occur.

These are the kinds of things MCOs will ask for in their application packet. By creating a concise statement about your practice, sometimes you can get your request for a provider application through the initial screening process.

Getting on Panels

Panels go through contracting phases when they are starting up, downsizing, or expanding. You will find the start-ups and expansion times in MCO publications, by networking with colleagues, reading the MCO publications you subscribe to, and through the use of MCO consultants. The best time to get into the system is when it is starting up. Joining small start-up MCOs can be effective since often they eventually are bought up by the larger MCOs and you may then be integrated into the larger panel. To get on provider panels:

The best time to get into the system is when it is starting up.

- Contact the MCOs providing services in your area, and ask what their needs are.
- Network with colleagues and let them know about your specialties. You may offer a service they do not have, and they may ask the MCO they are working with to send their client to you for special services.
- Consider calls from potential clients who use an MCO you are not affiliated with as a potential reason to be included in that panel. Have inquirers inform their employer that they want to use your services and need for you to be included in the MCO's panel. This request can also be presented to their EAP, primary care physician, or union steward. With this much pressure, you may be included in the panel or at least receive outside panel treatment authorization, which begins your relationship with the MCO.
- Subscribe to the publications that list open panels. When you receive your monthly copy, act immediately. Mail or fax your practice

packet requesting an application. Complete the packet as soon as you receive it and follow up on a response.

Computerize your credentials.

- Computerize your credentials. Make a database of all your professional information so that you do not need to go searching for it every time you fill out an application. A national company, HSP Verified, Inc., verifies credentials of providers, holds that information in a data bank, and provides that information to MCOs. There is a fee to register. Contact them at (202) 783-1270.
- Offer case rates. A case rate is a flat fee you accept to treat a client. You are the case manager and sink or swim on how you manage the case.
- Fill a geographic need in the MCO's delivery system. You can set up a satellite office by subletting from a colleague.
- Ask about the MCO's training needs and offer free training to its staff to educate them in an area in which you have expertise.
- Offer to treat an underserved population.
- Offer short-term groups.
- Offer services for adolescents.
- Don't market services that are outside Axis I or on Axis II *DSM* diagnoses since they often are not covered.
- Take a case manager to lunch.
- Offer free aftercare groups.
- Offer free psychoeducational classes for managers.

Track your responses. You can reapproach the companies that do not respond after you do more research about the company's needs. When you receive an application packet, complete it immediately and return it by priority mail.

Staying on Panels

Maintaining a High Provider Profile. A provider profile is a report card on how you have performed in the managed care industry:

- Providers who get the highest number of referrals have received an "A."

- Providers who get some referrals or are listed in directories and get no referrals have a grade of "B."
- Providers who get no referrals but are not eliminated from lists for fear of possible litigation are graded "C."

Provider profiles measure:

1. Utilization or cost per client case.
2. Clinical outcomes or how well treatment goals were met.
3. Process performance or the quality of communication between the case manager and the provider.
4. Technical performance such as the use of targeted focal therapy.
5. Patient satisfaction with the therapist.

Client surveys provide information for numbers 2 and 5; case manager evaluations provide information for numbers 3 and 4. Number 1 is measured by the utilization or average number of sessions per patient. The goal is to identify the most cost-effective and efficient providers.

Ways to Enhance Your Profile

- Be sensitive to the care manager's needs.
- Maintain a friendly relationship rather than an adversarial one.
- Be accessible and quickly responsive.
- Submit billing and reports in a timely manner.
- Think of yourself as being part of a team.
- Make treatment plans concrete and specific to the problem you are addressing. Include short- and long-term goals, and treatment interventions. Be clear about how you will help your client reach the treatment goals you have identified.
- Notify the case manager when new problems emerge or treatment is not going as you have planned (Lawless, 1997).
- Use electronic billing. More MCOs are moving to this form of billing. It is a win-win arrangement. It saves them time and money, and you get paid more promptly.

Make treatment plans concrete and specific to the problem you are addressing.

Outcome Measures

How can you convince an MCO you are a good provider? Use outcome measurement tools and complete a practice survey annually to report how good you are. The profile should include the level of psychiatric symptoms, clinical functioning, and patient satisfaction.

Patient satisfaction has been the driving factor in provider referrals. The MCO asks these kinds of questions:

- How quickly did the provider return your call?
- Were they courteous when you spoke to them?
- Was the information they gave you accurate?
- How promptly did they schedule an appointment?
- How easy was it to get to the provider's office?
- Was the office comfortable, safe, and clean?
- How well did the provider understand your problem and address your needs?
- Was the provider caring and concerned about your problems?

This information may not seem as important to you as your clinical expertise, but it most certainly matters to the MCO. In terms of clinical measures, short-term measures are best focused on symptom assessment, and long-term measures on functional assessment. The MCO is most interested in how strategically you addressed the problem and returned the client to functionality.

Planning to Work with MCOs

We recommend the following procedure for entering the MCO niche market. Complete the self-assessment at the beginning of this chapter and clarify your experiences with and beliefs about managed care. Identify the stage and phase of MCO development in your region. After you choose the type of MCO you want to target, decide which services and products you want to offer MCOs. Think about the special features of your practice that would entice an MCO to send you referrals. Next, complete a practice profile. If there are any topics that you do not have in place, make a plan for implementation. Explore your network to find out what MCOs are coming to your region, and subscribe to MCO publications to stay apprised of the field. After obtaining a list of MCOs offering services in your region, determine what action items you want to accomplish to get on local panels. Setting up an outcomes measurement system for your practice will enable you to regularly review what you are doing to ensure a high provider profile. Finally, complete an annual practice assessment and send it to MCOs.

Most MCOs prefer that you have an external office. If your office is in your home, observe the following criteria. Your office needs to have a separate entrance for your clients. That means they don't walk in your front door and have to step over the dog and the kids on the way to your office. Your office must look professional and be separate from the rest of the house. You can't use your dining room, even though you cleaned off the table. If clients need to use a bathroom, it must be for your office use only, and if clients have to wait, you need a designated waiting room, not your living room. Your home office needs to have its own telephone line. Also, check out the local business and zoning ordinances, and make sure you have insurance coverage for business liabilities.

Employee Assistance Programs (EAPs)

The stresses and demands in the workplace have helped create a growing need for EAP services. They have grown from 450 nationally in 1970 to more than 20,000 today. In the 1940s, the first EAPs were designed to deal with employees who were alcoholics. Today's EAPs have a wider scope of services and are a growing force in the healthcare industry. Employers who want to reduce the need for the use of an MCO often put them in place. EAPs can offer consultations, assessment, counseling, or referral services. EAPs often offer help with financial, substance abuse, or older parent problems. Some have in-house professionals and many use either an informal or formal external provider panel. Often an employee will first be referred to the EAP for a limited number of sessions (3–5), and when their EAP benefit is exhausted, they must draw on their other mental health benefits. This can be a problem if the client develops a therapeutic relationship during those first five visits and then has to be transferred to another clinician because their mental health plan will

Today's employee assistance programs have a wider scope of services and are a growing force in the healthcare industry.

not reimburse the clinician under contract with the EAP, or the EAP requires a change in provider.

Professionals who like to limit their practice to brief treatment or assessments enjoy working with EAPs. EAPs are also a good place for exposure to a company. You can contact the EAP coordinator and ask about their needs and whether you can make their job easier. If they do not already have wellness seminars in place, ask if you can present in-house psychoeducational programs for their employees during lunch. If they already have an educational staff, see if any topics are lacking and offer those. Presenting programs allows employees to get to know you; then when they use their mental health benefits, they will look for you. If you are not on their MCO panel, they may ask for you to be included. There are many videotapes that promote wellness, such as the videotapes prepared by the *Drug-Free Catalog* (800) 453-7733. Their videotapes are well produced and include skill-building guides. Another source is the EAP Association (703) 522-6272. When you become a member, you will receive the *EAP Digest*. It is an excellent publication and will keep you up to date on areas of need. Topics of interest for EAPs include but are not restricted to:

Workplace violence	Change management
Drug and alcohol abuse	Marital and relationship problems
Crisis prevention	Parenting
Aging parents	Stress and anxiety management
Grief	Recognizing a life problem
Codependency	Lifestyle change
Financial health	When executives need help
Legal problems	Dealing with diversity in the workplace

This niche market is also a good target for interactive computer training programs.

Many new workplace issues are emerging. A business publication that addresses the humanistic side of business is *Business Spirit Journal* (505) 474-0998; their latest issue discussed setting boundaries and having fun in the workplace. Stay on the leading edge but be careful of offering too many nontraditional treatment approaches.

Some strategies for getting referrals from EAPs include:

- *Write an introductory letter.* State briefly why you are qualified to provide services. Include a copy of your practice profile and your brochure and newsletter. When you list services, also include their cost. Include a current resume that has been designed to be of interest to an EAP.
- *Call and follow up on your letter and try to schedule an interview.* Some will want to meet you, and others might conduct an interview over the phone. The personal interview is preferable. During the interview, be a good listener and try to get an understanding of the company culture and the kind of employees they serve. Dress in appropriate business attire. Mental health counselors often wear more casual clothing than the general business community. For this interview, match their corporate culture.
- After your interview, follow up with periodic reminders that you are still available and send copies of your current newsletter.
- When you get a referral, call or send a note thanking them. Let them know when an appointment has been scheduled.
- Do not put a client on disability without referring back to the EAP.
- If they send you a provider manual, read it and ask questions if anything is unclear.
- When you are nearing the end of treatment, let the EAP know.
- When you terminate a client, send a termination summary.

Be a good listener and try to get an understanding of the company culture and the kind of employees they serve.

Other strategies to becoming more informed about this niche market are to explore EAP Provider Certification through EAPA and join your professional associations EAP special interest group.

Planning

Your plan will be different for whatever stage of preparedness you are in. The EAP mindmap shown in Figure 7.1 is a strategic plan with goals for start up, maintenance, and expansion phases of MCO involvement.

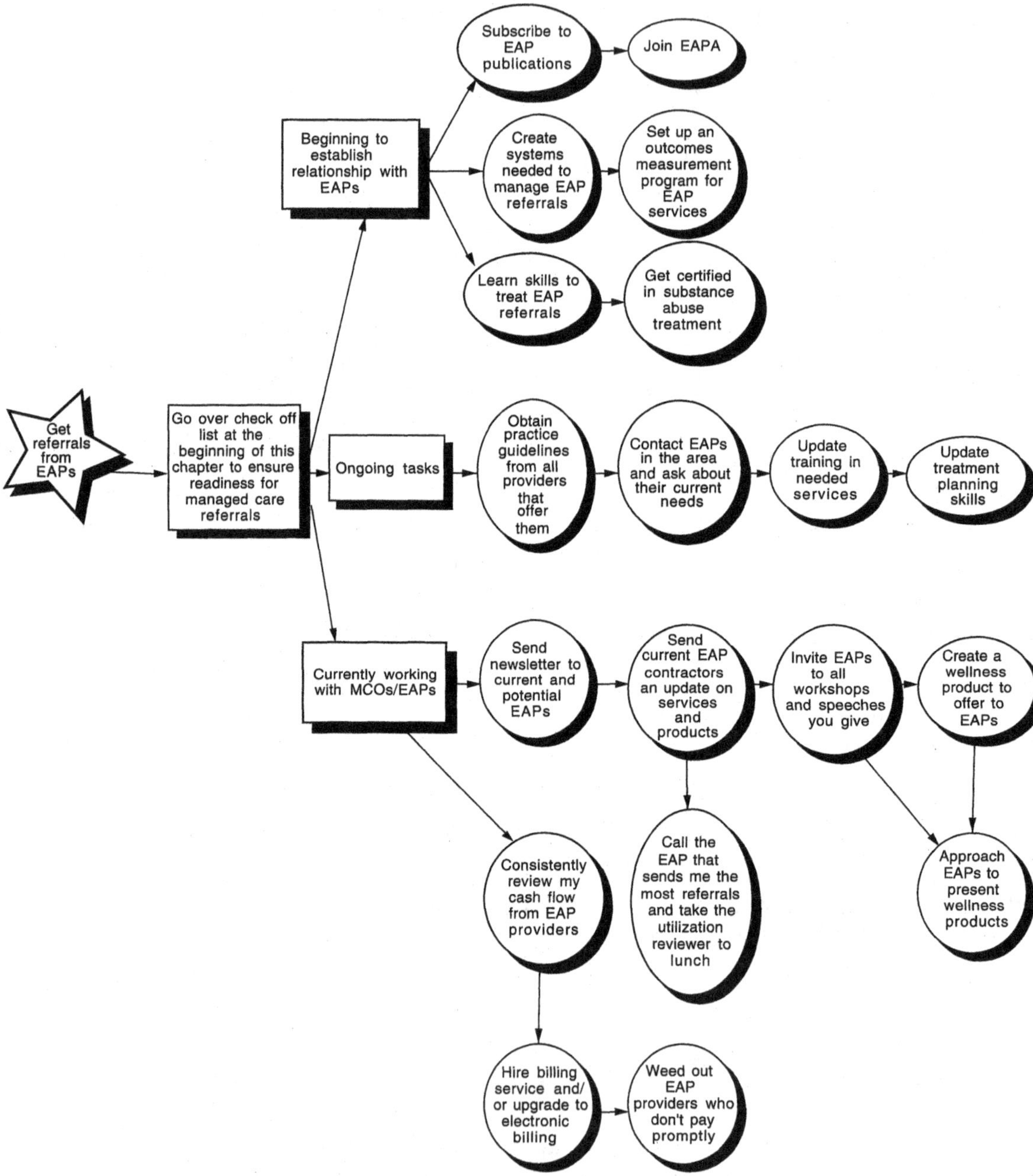

FIGURE 7.1 An EAP Mindmap

Outreach Vehicles

Advertisement

Many MCOs and EAPs, as well as the Employee Assistance Professional Association, have periodical publications. The *EAP Digest* (1270 Rankin Drive, Suite F, Troy MI 48083) has a Services Directory. You can place a 3.5 × 4 inch ad and be included in the Reader Service Card. Readers simply fill in the return card and automatically receive more information about your services. You can also place your ad in your local Yellow Pages under Employee Assistance Programs or any other heading in your area that is appropriate.

Newsletters

Newsletters need to be simple and easy to read. The topics must be relevant to the MCO and EAP market. Newsletters can be client-oriented or directed to the MCO or EAP staff member. The first newsletter in this chapter covers a treatment issue and could be given to a potential client.

The next brochure is directed to the MCO or EAP staff person. This newsletter is intended to help them remember your practice so when they make referrals, your name comes quickly to mind.

When your newsletters look professional, you can sell them to EAPs for their employees. There are already many in the marketplace and sometimes local EAPs like to use a local professional's materials. Charge a fair price and keep your series alive by adding timely topics. Check out the brochures and posters offered by the American Institute for Preventive Medicine at http://aipm.healthy.net/eap/index.html, or contact the Health Sentry at (800) 453-7733.

Directory Worksheet

As you gather information about MCOs and EAPs, maintain Practice Resource Directory worksheets about them. We keep ours in a database so that when we are looking for a particular resource we can search easily on the computer. A sample of a basic worksheet is shown in Figure 7.2.

Date: ____________ New: ________ Revision: ________

Name: ____

Address: ____

Organization: ____

Telephone(s): ____

Fax: ____________________ E-mail Address: ________________

Web site: ____

Contact Person: ____

Application Process: ____

Credentials Required: ____

Reimbursement: ____

Region Served: ____

Companies Served: ____

Needs, i.e., geographical areas underserved; specialities sought: ________________

Treatment Protocols Provided: ____

Notes:

Contact Dates and People:

Source: Adapted from L. Lawless *Therapy Inc.* (New York: John Wiley, 1997). Reprinted with permission.

FIGURE 7.2 Resource Directory Worksheet

Letters

Keep your outreach letters short and specific. Start with who you are and where your practice is located. Let them know about your experience with managed care, which could include working in a community mental health agency. Emphasize your adherence to an MCO-friendly approach (strategic, symptom-oriented treatment). Your resume needs to be equally short, no more than two pages. The sample shown in Figure 7.3 uses the recommended format.

Fax-Back Sheet

Since you are dealing with businesses and not individuals, a fax-back sheet (Figure 7.4) can be used in place of the return card. This means you need to have a dedicated fax line. If an EAP or MCO wants to send you a fax and it does not go through, they may not try again. You can include any information you want checked off on your sheet.

Since you are dealing with businesses and not individuals, a fax-back sheet can be used in place of the return card.

Brochure

You can use three kinds of brochures for this niche market: your practice brochure, informational brochures, and informational brochures for MCO and EAP staff.

Telephone Script

You are more likely to reach a decision maker in an Employee Assistance Program than a large Managed Care Organization. The telephone script on pages 228–229 is oriented toward a mid-sized EAP. The script is a guide for directing the conversation.

To Do List

A simple "To Do" list facilitates accountability and helps you use your time wisely (see page 230).

Alpha Centre

6 Pleasant Street Suite 214 Malden MA 02148 781-322-3051

Our mission is to be a professional resource in support of the health and well-being of

- *The whole person*
- *Families*
- *Businesses, institutions, and*
- *Municipalities*

in the service of creating caring community

Our services include psychoeducational workshops on:

EATING DISORDERS

DRUG & ALCOHOL ABUSE

UNRESOLVED GRIEF

PARENTING TRAINING

COMMUNICATION SKILLS AND CONFLICT MANAGEMENT

STRESS REDUCTION

SUCCESSFUL MEDIATION

CO-DEPENDENCY

SURVIVING AND THRIVING AS A STEP-FAMILY

CAREER CHANGE

MENTAL ILLNESS WHAT IS IT?

SUCCESSFUL AGING

SUCCESSFUL LIFESTYLE CHANGE

Dear Provider Relations Department *(It is best to call ahead and get the name of the Provider Relations Staff member you are directing the letter to)*

I am interested in becoming a mental health provider for ___________ (insert name of company). In my Boston, MA office, which is wheelchair accessible and close to public transportation. I provide services for individuals, couples and families. My office provides a confidential and safe environment for clients with plenty of parking in a well lit parking lot.

I currently work with local EAPs and managed care firms who seem to be pleased with my quality of care and strategic, solution focused treatment philosophy. I use a practice management system that ensures prompt electronic billing and clear, timely, and concise treatment plans and reports. I also have an outcomes program in place and can provide bi-annual reports or reports on-demand at any time.

I am enclosing a more detailed practice profile that covers my specialities, i.e., alcohol and substance abuse, eating disorders and more. I am also sending a a copy of an informational newsletter I provide for clients and a LifeStyle newsletter I offer colleagues.

For your members convenience, I have evening and weekend hours available and can accommodate new clients within 36 hours.

Please send me a new provider packet or contact me if you have any additional questions. I have provided a convenient FAX back sheet for a more prompt response.

Sincerely,

FIGURE 7.3 Sample MCO Outreach Letter

Please FAX to The Alpha Centre @ 781.322.3051

Yes! Yes! Yes! ....I WANT TO KNOW MORE ABOUT THE ALPHA CENTRE

________*YES! PLEASE CALL ME AT THE NUMBER BELOW. I/MY ORGANIZATION IS INTERESTED IN YOUR SERVICES AND WOULD LIKE TO TALK DIRECTLY TO YOU.*

________*YES! PLEASE CALL ME AT THE NUMBER BELOW. I KNOW OF ANOTHER ORGANIZATION THAT WOULD BE INTERESTED IN YOUR SERVICES.*

________*YES! I WANT TO PURCHASE YOUR INFORMATIONAL BROCHURES, PLEASE SEND ME AN ORDER SHEET.*

________*YES! I WOULD LIKE TO RECEIVE YOUR FREE NEWSLETTER SO I MAY LEARN MORE ABOUT HOW YOUR SERVICES CAN HELP ME AND MY ORGANIZATION GROW AND IMPROVE. I HAVE LISTED MY CONTACT INFORMATION BELOW:*

Your Name and Address:

Name: ________________________________

Title: ________________________________

Company: ________________________________

Address: ________________________________

____

Telephone: ________________________________

FAX: ________________________________

E-mail: ________________________________

Comments: ________________________________

____

IF YOU PREFER, MAIL TO THE ALPHA CENTRE
@ 6 PLEASANT STREET, SUITE 214, MALDEN MA 02148
OR CALL US AT 781.322.3051

FIGURE 7.4 Fax-Back Sheet

Telephone Script

Preparing. The EAP manager has received your letter and brochures in advance:

- Have a copy of the materials in front of you.
- Have some knowledge of the company or companies the EAP provides services for. Know the name of the administrator who is in charge of provider services.
- Call when you are feeling refreshed and confident.
- Be prepared to not make contact on the first call; do not hesitate to call back.
- Be prepared to focus and take charge of the call since EAP managers are busy professionals.
- Take a deep breath and place the call.

Connecting:

- You reach the receptionist or secretary. Identify yourself and your practice and ask to speak with the administrator. Share that you are responding to his or her request for information if the mail-back card has been returned. If not, say that you are calling to discuss your mailing with him or her. If you know a person in common, let the receptionist or secretary know that they have referred or recommended the EAP professional to you. You will most likely receive a high priority. If he or she is not available, ask that your call be returned, leaving your telephone number with times you may be reached. If you do not receive a return call within a day or two, do not hesitate to call again. Remember that administrators are busy professionals. Create a follow-up note to call again.
- You reach the EAP administrator. Have your script in hand and follow it. Keep your text to one page and remember that the call is about building a relationship. In your first paragraph, you begin building the relationship. Introduce yourself and your business; mention that you are a licensed mental health professional:

  "This is ______, of ______. I'm a licensed ______ and have been practicing in (name of community) since ______. "

[If you know someone who knows the EAP professional, mention the person's name and your relationship to him or her at this time. Let this person know that you will be calling the EAP administrator.]

Presentation. This comprises the second paragraph and contains your reason for calling:

> "Did you receive the letter and brochure I mailed on ______ ? Do you have questions, comments about it?"

Share why you want to work with EAPs (your particular areas of specialties which correlate with the EAP's needs) and that you believe that you share mutual interests, which can benefit you both.

- Ask how long has this EAP been providing employee services. How did you come to work in an EAP? What special needs do your EAP employees have? Who do you use for direct employee services, in-house psychoeducational events, or psychoeducational products? Be interested and keep your questions specific to the topic.
- Ask if they have worked with outside mental health professionals before. Mention services, products, or educational topics you have that their in-house or current outside professionals may not have. You may also base comments on your mission statement. Invite the administrator's ideas about common ground. For example, employees who are going through a divorce and include comments about your training and experience in the field. Share that you are respectful of confidentiality issues. This will aid in building the bridges of trust and openness with them. For example: Have you worked with mental health professionals before? If so, what has been your experience?
- Ask if there are regular meetings of EAP administrators (a local EAPA) you might be invited to. If so, to whom would you speak to about the possibility of attending? Offer yourself as a speaker on a topic of interest to them. Can he or she be helpful or is there another contact? If so, who is the person you should speak to?

Close. The third paragraph brings closure to the telephone meeting. If all has gone well and you feel that there is a like-minded interest, invite the EAP administrator to lunch or ask for an appointment to meet and further discuss how you might assist one another. Make appropriate thank yous and close with a "looking forward to meeting you in person" statement.

Affirming. Give yourself a pat on the back! You're on your way to building a niche market.

Completing. Follow up the telephone call with a note stating that you appreciate the time taken and that you look forward to the possibility of working together around your common interests in the future. If you have scheduled a luncheon meeting and/or appointment to meet, mention it.

To Do List

- Look in the Yellow Pages under Employee Assistance Programs and select those who serve the kinds of people you would work with effectively (i.e., professional, construction, hotel, or restaurant).
- Obtain a copy of the Employee Assistance Professionals Association's local directory and do the same as above.
- Check the EAPA web site for local EAP providers by [date].
- List names of friends, family, and colleagues who might be able to supply names of EAPs or EAP professionals or administrators. [Date] you will call them.
- Call [date].
- Prepare mailing to those who match with your skills and resources by [date].
- Develop brochure by [date].
- Write cover letters by [date].
- Develop and write enclosures by [date].
- Develop and write newsletter by [date].
- Mail packet by [date].
- Schedule calling date.
- Prepare and review your telephone script and practice aloud.
- Integrate all dates with your Goals Plan.
- Mail thank-you note by [date]. Here is a sample letter:

  Dear _______:

  It was a pleasure to learn about your EAP program. I enjoyed speaking with you and appreciated your time taken. Because we both work with people who are having mental or emotional difficulties, it is good to have a resource in the mental health field for referrals. I look forward to future contact with you. Please do not hesitate to contact me if you have further questions.

Summary

The managed care marketplace is complex and challenging. Those who embrace it and work well in it can flourish in their profession. The marketplace continues to change. If you choose to work here, stay informed and never get too comfortable with any referral source. The key words here are caution and perseverance.

Resources

Associations

Employee Assistance Professionals Association (EAPA) directory—(703) 387-1000

Employee Assistance Society of North America (EASNA)—(312) 644-0828

Conferences

Managed Behavioral Healthcare Conference—(800) 345-8016

National Managed Health Care Congress—(617) 487-6700

Institute for Behavioral Healthcare—(415) 851-6469

North American Congress on EAPs (NAC/EAP)—(313) 643-9580

Employee Assistance Professionals Association (EAPA) Annual Conference—(703) 387-1000

Credentialing

Certified Employee Assistance Professional (CEAP)—is provided through EAPA.

Glossaries

Tuttle, G.M. (1994). *The Managed Care Sourcebook*. Washington, DC: AAMFT.

Browning, C.H., & Browning, B.J. (1994). *How to Partner with Managed Care*. Los Alamitos, CA: Duncliff's International.

Internet

Interpsych is a newsletter you can subscribe to online. Send e-mail to listserv@fra.psych.nemc.org and in the body of the e-mail type "subscribe."

Lists of MCOs—EAPA www.EAP-Association.com/

Mental Health Associates—www.mentalhealth_madison.com

MCO/EAP Lists

National Association of Insurance Commissioners—www.naic.org

Your Professional Association (i.e., American Psychiatric Association; American Psychological Association; National Association of Social Workers; American Association of Marriage Family Therapists; American Mental Health Counselors Association; American Counseling Association)

Tuttle, G.M. (1994). *The Managed Care Sourcebook.* Washington, DC: AAMFT.

Outcome Measures

Basis-32 (617) 855-2425 McLean Hospital

SF-35 (617) 426-4046 Medical Outcomes Trust

SCR-90-R Symptom Checklist (800) 627-7271 National Computer Systems

Periodicals

Psychotherapy Finances (800) 869-8450

Behavioral Healthcare Tomorrow (415) 435-9821

Open Minds (717) 334-1329

Practice Management Monthly (800) 578-5013

Managed Care Strategies (800) 869-8450

EAP Digest (703) 522-6272

Business Spirit Journal (505) 474-0998

Training Aids

EAP Association (703) 522-6272

CompreCare Publishers: 2415 Annappolis Lane, Suite 140, Minneapolis, MN 55441

Hazelton: Pleasant Valley Road, Box 176, Center City, MN 55012

Recommended Reading

Ackley, D.C. (1997). *Breaking free of managed care: A step-by-step guide to regaining control of your practice.* New York: Guilford Press.

Browning, C.H., & Browning, B.J. (1994). *How to partner with managed care.* New York: Duncliff's International.

Davis, J. (Ed.). (1996). *Marketing for therapists.* New York: Jossey-Bass.

Ginter, E.J., Kelly, E.R., & Lawless, L.L. (1998). *Managed care: What mental health counselors need to know*. An unpublished paper.

Marketing: A guide to unmanaged care. (1996). *Practice Management Monthly*, 4(2), 6.

Miller, I. (1994). *What managed care is doing to outpatient mental health*. Boulder, CO: Boulder Psychotherapy Press.

Poynter, W. (1994). *The preferred provider's handbook*. New York: Brunner/Mazel.

Tuckfelt, S., Fink, J., & Warren, M.P. (1997). *The psychotherapists' guide to managed care in the 21st century*. New Jersey: Jason Aronson.

8

Strategies for Marketing to Mental Health and Complementary Healthcare Professionals

To achieve a thriving, successful, meaningful private practice, the mental health professional must be a bridge-builder to other professional groups. Today's marketplace smiles on collegiality, diversity, team building, and the sharing of information rather than the competition, elitism, and protectiveness so inherent in marketplace dynamics of earlier decades. We see the remnants of this divisiveness in the competition for market share by different license categories (e.g., psychologists, social workers, professional counselors, marriage/family therapists).

This divisiveness emerges out of the evolution of the professions and ways in which the modern professional has been trained. The word *profession* originally applied to the vows taken by those who entered into religious life. The word has come to mean any vocation that embodies a particular field of knowledge, such as medicine or law. Today, the term *profession* has expanded to include a huge number of work venues, particularly those areas that have developed graduate or specialized training programs for practitioners with standards and avenues for entry into the field.

Specialized graduate programs tend to distance professionals from engagement with other professional disciplines and with the communities in which they practice because turf and resource/money battles have raised strong boundaries around each graduate school. As a result, trainees have had little dialogue with other professional groups and limited input from those who need the professional services. This dynamic facilitated an "expert (the professional)—uneducated laity (the buyer of services)" dichotomy. In this era of the responsible and educated consumer, this model is rapidly losing relevancy. On the ascendancy is a model that engages the professional and the consumer as co-responsible co-learners.

Not only is staying in touch with your potential referral markets a marketing issue, it is a social issue. Thomas Bender, writing in the *Kettering Review* (Winter 1994), differentiates two paradigms: "civic professionalism" and "disciplinary professionalism." The civic professionalism paradigm is descriptive of a time prior to the industrial age when community leaders in cities such as Florence, Italy, practiced what Mr. Bender calls *civic humanism*. These leaders practiced their professional expertise while also actively serving the community by supporting the building of libraries, museums, hospitals, schools, and other institutions that enhanced life for all community members.

Not only is staying in touch with your potential referral markets a marketing issue, it is a social issue.

Practitioners of this style of civic professionalism include men and women like Florence Nightingale, founder of the profession of nursing; Jane Addams, founder of neighborhood centers that served the needs of immigrants; and Samuel Bard, M.D., one of the founders of the New York Hospital in 1771. These civic professionals and others like them were actively engaged in community life, enhancement of the welfare of all members of the community, and the intellectual dialogue of the community.

Mr. Bender uses the term disciplinary professionalism to describe a paradigm shift that arose out of the industrial age and cultural change of the nineteenth century and evoked a unique form or expression of professionalism. This model viewed professionals as related to a branch of science, a discipline, rather than as professionals connected or related to a civic role: ". . . each new disciplinary profession developed its own conceptual basis as evidenced by the development of graduate training schools. Each became a distinct 'epistemic community'" (p. 50).

Mr. Bender wonders if the disciplinary professional paradigm is helpful in light of current realities, changes, and needs in civic life. He quotes Alfred North Whitehead on the subject:

> Each professional makes progress, but it is progress in its own groove. But there is no groove . . . adequate for the comprehension of human life. . . . Of course, no one is merely a mathematician, or merely a lawyer. People have lives outside of their profession or their business. But the point is the restraint of serious thought within a groove. The remainder of life is treated superficially, with the imperfect categories of thought derived from one profession.

Most of today's mental health practitioners have been trained in the disciplinary professionalism model. Dialoguing with students in other professional schools of thought was often ignored, or worse, discouraged. Loyalty was to one's own school and categories of thought. Now there is a slow shift toward inviting professionals to move out of the "groove" and engage in dialogue between various professional schools.

Such dialogue is positive and indicative of paradigm shifts taking place in business and the professions as we explore the uncertainties and unpredictability of the Information Age, and the healthcare market. A synthesis of these two models is urgently needed for you to have a thriving mental health professional practice. You must bridge the two models—civic professional and disciplinary professional—in a way that allows you to creatively move across these disciplinary professional boundaries. Not only has the disciplinary professional model inhibited cross-disciplinary connection, it has often isolated the mental health practitioner from the civic life of the community. A civic-minded mental health professional who is committed to developing connections with mental healthcare practitioners across the disciplinary boundaries will survive and thrive in today's marketplace. Sam Conant, a clinical social worker in Vermont was quoted in *Practice Strategies* (August 1998):

A civic-minded mental health professional who is committed to developing connections with mental healthcare practitioners across the disciplinary boundaries will survive and thrive in today's marketplace.

> Community involvement is the key to a successful business and life. . . . Volunteer work is useful. And though that's not why you do it, it can also be good for your practice. For example, I volunteered to help during the terrible ice storm we had last winter—getting people to shelter, delivering food, providing transportation, etc. I ended up getting over 25 referrals as a result of people I met and worked with during that time. (pp. 7–8)

Holding a systemic model enables you to bridge the civic and disciplinary paradigms. Envisioning yourself as one element connecting to and relating with many other mental health practitioners in your location enhances and nurtures your practice. A synthesis of the civic and the disciplinary is a necessity for a viable practice. This systemic model enables you to have a sense of yourself as an important component not only in the local mental health well-being of the community, but also in the larger regional, national, and global system of behavioral healthcare and mental well-being. This model embraces community mental health workers, those in private practice, in hospital settings, in school settings, and so on. It includes those who are credentialed differently than yourself as well as complementary healthcare professionals and others in the human service field.

Values that support the necessity of cooperation between professional practitioners are not unique. The February 1997 issue of *Family Therapy News* reported that 10 national health and mental health organizations collaborated on a Bill of Rights to protect those seeking treatment for mental illness and/or psychological disorders. The Bill of Rights was a response to their perception that people are not being well served in the current healthcare system. The 10 collaborators were supported in their effort by three lay organizations: National Alliance for the Mentally Ill, National Mental Health Association, and the National Depressive and Manic-Depressive Association. This is an example of bridging civic and disciplinary interests.

Such an alignment of the leadership in these influential professional and lay national groups likely aided passage of the 1998 Mental Health Parity Act, which provides for parity between mental health and medical/surgical benefits. Although it is yet to be seen how parity will work, 19 states have passed similar legislation; 13 more states are pending. Collaboration and collegiality can be highly beneficial at every level of the social web.

Because mental health practitioners are part of the overall system, consider them as another group to which you can market your services/products. Develop a strategic marketing plan for them as well as for complementary or alternative healthcare providers related to this field. Envision practicing in a different groove.

Because mental health practitioners are part of the overall system, consider them as another group to which you can market your services/products.

Characteristics of Mental Health Practitioners

An article in the *Family Therapy News*, "How MFTs Compare to Other Disciplines," (April 1997, p. 17) pointed out that except for psychiatry, which has a majority of older men, women compose the greatest number of mental health professionals. According to the following statistics, psychology and marriage and family therapy have more gender balance within their particular specialties:

- Counselors—78 percent female; 22 percent male.
- Marriage and family therapists—53 percent female; 47 percent male.
- Psychiatric nursing—95 percent female; 5 percent male.
- Psychiatry—25 percent female; 75 percent male.
- Psychology—44 percent female; 56 percent male.
- Psychosocial rehabilitation—not available.
- School psychology—not available.
- Social work—77 percent female; 23 percent male.
- Complementary healthcare professionals—not available.

The following data are for professionals with 10 years in practice:

- Counselors—15.8 percent.
- Marriage and family therapists—61.5 percent.
- Psychiatric nursing—58.6 percent.
- Psychiatry—86.7 percent.
- Psychology—61.2 percent.
- Psychosocial rehabilitation—78.2 percent.
- School psychology—52.6 percent.
- Social work—54.9 percent.
- Complementary healthcare professionals—not available.

In terms of ethnic participation in the various mental health groups, data revealed the following:

- Counselors—data not available.
- Marriage and family therapists—4.8 percent of males and 3.3 percent of females are of minority groups, with the largest group being American Indian; the next largest ethnic group is American Indian/Alaska Native.
- Psychiatric nursing—9.3 percent of males and 4.0 percent of females are of minority groups. The largest percentage are African American followed by Hispanic or American Indian/Alaska Native.

- Psychiatry—21 percent of females and 13.7 percent of males are from minorities with the largest percentage being Asian/Pacific Islander.
- Psychology— 7.2 percent of females and 5.3 percent of males are primarily Hispanic or African American.
- Psychosocial rehabilitation—30.2 percent of the males are primarily African American; data not available for females.
- School psychology— 6.4 percent of females and 6 percent of males are primarily African American or Hispanic.
- Social work—9.9 percent of females and 9.7 percent of males are primarily African American or Hispanic.
- Complementary healthcare professionals—data not available.

These characteristics suggest that as you prepare to deepen your connections with colleagues in the mental health arena, you most often will be relating to white women with several years of clinical experience. In your network building, you need to pursue ethnic diversity with diligence. At a minimum, seek diversity of theoretical schools and licensures/certifications, including the complementary professionals. A large number of them are in private practice (see under The Marketplace). Private practitioners often need to develop additional skills and creativity to continue in the work that gives them meaning and purpose. This may be an area in which you could develop a niche market.

In your network building, you need to pursue ethnic diversity with diligence.

Alternative Healthcare Providers

The complementary/alternative healing modalities have been around since the beginning of recorded history. In the beginning of civilization, they would have been the only healing modality available. Recently, there has been a resurgence of interest in alternative healthcare as people have learned more about the Oriental healing arts, particularly meditation, visioning, and acupuncture. Lynette Bassman's book *The Whole Mind: The Definitive Guide to Complementary Treatments for Mind, Mood, and Emotion* (1998) provides a description of thirty-six complementary healthcare categories along with organizations and resources for further learning.

Five basic concepts common to complementary practitioners are:

Allopathic medicine follows the Western, germ/virus understanding of illness and disease.

Preventive medicine is the best medicine.

1. Psychosomatic versus somatopsychic refers to the understanding that mind/body—body/mind is interactive, integrated, reciprocal, and functions as a single unit.
2. Allopathic and holistic describe two methods of providing healthcare. Allopathic medicine follows the Western, germ/virus understanding of illness and disease. It is the medical, scientific method and treats "parts" of the body with specialties for those parts. Allopathic medicine has been practiced for about one hundred years. Holistic, which predates the allopathic, takes a preventive as well as treatment stance and points again to the fully integrated aspect of the body/mind system. Followers of this approach believe that all parts of the human system work together to maintain health.
3. The body functions to heal itself. Give the body time to heal instead of interfering with inherent healing properties (e.g., if there is a toxin in the system, the body cleanses itself via fever, vomiting, and/or diarrhea). Part of a holistic healer's expertise has to do with knowing when to intervene, and to what degree, and when to allow bodily processes to manage the healing.
4. Cumulative stress lessens the body's ability to recover. Stress is ubiquitous and includes mental, emotional, and physical stressors; it is an essential, inevitable element of life. Disease results when the body/mind is no longer able to mediate the stressors. Reducing the stress/stressors allows the body/mind to marshal its inherent healing mechanisms.
5. Preventive medicine is the best medicine. Conditions are best treated at a subtle rather than full-blown stage. Holistic healing styles often include techniques for enhancing awareness of imbalances. Imbalance can be dealt with prior to a disease manifesting.

Our clients often ask us about complementary healthcare practices and we need to be, at minimum, informed enough to respond and/or offer resources on the topic. How many clients have asked you about St. John's Wort, the herbal medicine suggested as a remedy for depression? Or maybe they asked you about Kava, an herbal medicine used to combat anxiety. The following list* of 53 complementary health modalities provides a definition for each:

Acupressure: The application of pressure to acupuncture points for treatment of asthma, back pain, childhood illnesses, fatigue, headache, and joint problems.

Acupuncture: Fine needles inserted into the body to improve health. Often used to treat allergies, anxiety, back pain, childhood illnesses, digestive disorders, eye disorders, headaches, insomnia, joint problems, labor pains, menstrual imbalances, mental and emotional problems, migraine, morning sickness, sinusitis, tinnitus, and more.

Alexandar technique: Therapy focused on balance and movement. Used for body tensions, headaches, and postural problems.

Aromatherapy: Plant oils for treatment of acne, anxiety, cellulite, colds, eczema, hay fever, headaches, indigestion, insect bites, premenstrual tension, postnatal depression, and skin conditions.

Autogenic training: Creative visualization and relaxation therapy in the treatment of AIDS, depression, eczema, fatigue, tension, high blood pressure, indigestion, insomnia, irritable bowel syndrome, and more.

Automatic Computerized Treatment System (ACTS): Computerized radionic programs that treat disease by measuring and analyzing energy patterns.

Ayurveda: Treatment for arthritis, diabetes, stress, ulcers, and other diseases, Ayurveda is the traditional medicine of India and focuses on the mind/body, spirit/soul balance.

Bach flower remedies: Flower essences used for mental/emotional disorders, anxiety, depression, and other illnesses.

Bates method: Relaxation exercises for eye disorders such as glaucoma and squint.

Biochemic tissue salts: Tissue salts used to treat aching feet and legs, brittle nails, colic, coughs, hair loss, hay fever, heartburn,

*This feature is reprinted with permission from Terri Ramacus, a Guide at About.com, Inc. About.com, Inc. can be found on the Web at www.about.com. To follow this series online at Terri Ramacus's site on Alternative Medicine at About.com, go to http://altmedicine.about.com.

muscular pain, rheumatic conditions, sciatica, sinus disorders, varicose veins, and so on.

Bioenergetics: Integration of body/mind in treating asthma, migraine, ulcers, and stress-related disorders.

Biofeedback: Relaxation therapy via technological help. Used in treating high blood pressure, anxiety, stress, and migraines.

Biorhythms: Used in treating depression and other general health conditions. Physical, intellectual, and emotional cycles are identified as an aid to understanding individual behavior.

Bowen technique: Use of balance and movement through creative arts therapy.

Celloid minerals: Treatment of anemia, diarrhea, goiter, high blood pressure, infertility, kidney stones, osteoporosis, premenstrual syndrome with minerals.

Chi Kung: Development of internal energy for treatment of many health conditions.

Chinese herbal medicine: Treatment with Chinese herbs and herbal extracts used in a wide variety of health conditions.

Chiropractic: Often used for treating back pain, headaches, joint sprains, muscular pain, sciatica, stiffness, and tennis elbow via joint manipulation.

Colonic irrigation: Hydrotherapy of the colon often used as part of a detoxification program and to treat candida.

Cranial osteopathy: Manipulation of the bones of the skull, used for childbirth pains, ADD, ADHD, learning difficulties, sinus conditions, temporomandibular joint (TMJ), and tinnitus.

Craniosacral therapy (CST): An adaptation of cranial osteopathy.

Creative art therapy: The use of the arts as a form of therapy. Used in behavioral problems, headaches, stress, some skin problems.

Cupping: Suction cups to remove impure energy from the body.

Dream work: Using dream recall to treat emotional illnesses such as depression.

Environmental therapies: Used to treat health conditions such as allergies and eczema, which may be caused by environmental conditions.

Feldenkrais: A movement therapy often used to treat arthritis, back pain, stress, and tension.

Feng Shui: Chinese practice of balancing energies in dwellings.

Hellerwork: Focuses on realignment of body to improve health and used for stress, tension, and posture.

Herbal medicine: Medicines derived from herbs. Used for many health conditions.

Homeopathy: Natural remedies used to boost the body's healing ability. Used in many situations.

Hydrotherapy: Water used therapeutically and applicable to labor pain and childbirth, muscle problems, rheumatism, stress, and tension.

Hypnotherapy: Enhances healing and well-being. Used to treat phobias and to change behavior patterns/habits.

Light therapy: Used to treat such conditions as seasonal affective disorder and depression.

Magnetic therapy: Rebalancing bodily energy to facilitate healing.

Massage: Relaxation of the body and use of touch to encourage healing and well-being.

Metamorphic technique: Physical and mental problems treated by manipulation of the foot.

Moxibustion: Application of heat to acupuncture joints. Used in many health conditions as well as childbirth.

Myotherapy: Diffusion of trigger points in muscles to relieve pain and retrain muscles.

Naturopathy: Incorporation of diet, exercise, counseling, and other gentle methods for assisting the body in its healing ability. Used in the treatment of anxiety, arthritis, asthma, bacterial infections, bronchitis, colds, depression, fatigue, kidney problems, skin problems, and other conditions.

Oriental herbal medicine: Use of herbs for health, based on Eastern therapies. Used in a wide variety of health conditions.

Osteopathy: Manipulative therapy that treats skeletal problems. Used in back pain, aches and pains following childbirth, gynecological problems, sprains, reduced jaw mobility, sciatica, and sports injuries.

Polarity therapy: A method for balancing vital energy forces within the body.

Psychodrama: Feelings acted out as an emotional release (cf. creative arts therapy).

Radionics: The measurement and analyzing of energy patterns to diagnose and treat diseases.

Reflexology: Massage of reflex points on feet and hands to encourage well-being. Used to treat back pain, infertility, multiple sclerosis, sinusitis, headaches, and stress.

Reiki: "Attunements" of bodily energy used to address a wide variety of health conditions.

Rolfing: Tissues treated to improve posture and health.

Shamanism: A traditional spiritual medicine. The power of nature and the Divine are used to encourage healing.

Shiatsu: Stimulation of vital points along the body's meridians to facilitate healing and to maintain good health.

T'ai Chi: Life force energy in the body developed via a series of circular, slow movements. Used for general health issues.

Therapeutic touch: Use of the hands to facilitate healing.

Traditional Chinese medicine: Acupressure, acupuncture, cupping, moxibustion, and Chinese herbal medicine.

Yoga: Spiritual and physical exercises to encourage health and well-being. Used for anxiety, arthritis, headache, migraine, multiple sclerosis, osteoporosis, pregnancy, rheumatoid arthritis, and other conditions.

More than 30 medical schools now offer courses in alternative medicine including Harvard, Columbia, Stanford, and Georgetown University. A 1993 Harvard medical school study found that two-thirds of Americans had relied on some form of alternative medicine in the previous year. A September 1998 survey of 1,000 Americans by the Stanford University School of medicine found that 69 percent had used alternative therapy in the previous year—the majority for preventive reasons and usually while also seeing a medical doctor. This growing interest is a primary reason for forging networks and building bridges to complementary practitioners with whom you feel professionally comfortable.

The complementary healthcare field is complex with much divergence in licensing and credentialing. The most helpful avenue to locate practitioners is to check listings in your Yellow Pages. Also, contact state licensing agencies for information regarding any registering policies and mailing lists related to complementary healthcare practitioners. You may also check your local city hall for regulations that affect alternative healthcare practitioners such as massage therapist. You might attend and/or have a booth at a Whole Health Expo as a way to learn more about the field as well as connect with complementary healthcare practitioners.

Complementary/Alternative Healthcare is growing phenomenally and is gaining attention in the healthcare market.

Complementary/Alternative Healthcare is growing phenomenally and is gaining attention in the healthcare market. It therefore presents much potential and possibility for successful collaboration and cooperation. Seek out those with whom you most resonate. Although what follows may not always allude to complementary healthcare practitioners, the information is often pertinent to them.

The Marketplace

There are approximately 433,519 mental health practitioners in the United Strates (*Family Therapy News,* April 1997). In addition, there are also approximately 10,000 acupuncturists (medical and nonmedical). Numbers for other therapists in the complementary healthcare field are not available. The national baseline number of therapists you have as a potential market for products and services would be about 50 percent of the number since all therapists are not in private practice. Locally and regionally, the number available to you for building a referral network depends on several factors, including:

- Your state—numbers of mental health and complementary care practitioners.
- The location of your practice—rural, urban, or suburban.
- Your region—you may choose to add workshops and seminars to your outreach.
- The culture of your community/state/regions—openness to mental health practitioners.

See Figure 8.1 for a list of numbers of therapists per 100,000 population on a state-by-state basis, along with percentages of the population in managed care Medicaid.

Actuarial data say that the optimum ratio for therapists to population is 70 therapists per 100,000 population. As Figure 8.1 shows, only 13 states reflect such a ratio (Alabama, Arkansas, Georgia, Idaho, Iowa, Kentucky, Mississippi, Nebraska, Nevada, North Carolina, North Dakota, South Carolina, and South Dakota). All other states are over the ratio. States with the highest number of therapists to population are: Massachusetts, New York, Vermont, Connecticut, Maryland, California, New Mexico, Maine, and New Jersey and range from a high of 229 per 100,000 to 137 per 100,000. (Washington, DC, not a state, is first with 325 per 100,000.) The incursions of managed care, both in the public and private spheres, add additional stresses for the private practice mental health professional since they must be included on managed care provider panels to receive referrals. If you live in a state with a high number of therapists per 100,000 and a large percentage of citizens enrolled in managed care then you are in a precarious professional position.

For example, Massachusetts has 229 therapists for 100,000 population which is the second highest ratio in the nation. Such numbers are indicative of abundant opportunities for networking and outreach as well as of a field seriously overpopulated with therapists according to actuarial data. If therapists in Massachusetts look to managed care organizations as their *primary or sole* income source for clients and income, they may need to relocate. This type of information provides clues for the products/services you may develop into a niche market such as: practice development, expansion of one's market to create multiple income streams, and development of the therapist's businessperson self.

At this time, we are in the midst of a major professional crisis as medical and mental healthcare models shift nationally. One of every five mental health professionals is preparing to leave the field. The transition of mental health practitioners from one vocation to another may provide possibilities for niche market opportunities (for example, career counseling, transitioning dynamics, support group facilitation around career change).

You need to be resilient, creative, and innovative in developing your practice.

If there are more than 70 therapists per 100,000 population in your state, and a large number of citizens are enrolled in public and/or private managed care, then you need to be resilient, creative, and innovative in developing your practice. You must take the initiative in marketing your

Percent of Clinicians per 100,000 & Managed Care Medicaid per State 1997
(Practice Strategies, October 1997, p. 6)

State	Clinicians per 100,000	Percent of Managed Care Medicaid
U.S.	113.4	40.1%
AL	47.0	11.4
AK	141.5	0.0
AZ	81.8	86.1
AR	55.2	38.6
CA	138.5	23.1
CO	124.1	79.6
CT	143.8	61.3
DC	325.4	55.4
DE	72.5	77.6
FL	73.7	63.7
GA	64.1	32.0
HI	106.1	80.4
ID	68.6	36.7
IL	80.1	12.9
IN	80.4	31.3
IA	59.2	41.4
KS	77.9	31.7
KY	54.3	53.2
LA	76.3	5.6
ME	137.3	0.8
MD	138.8	63.5
MA	228.8	69.8
MI	125.0	72.7
MN	98.6	33.2
MS	32.1	6.9
MO	81.9	34.5
MT	99.5	59.4
NE	63.5	27.5
NV	61.9	40.9
NH	108.5	16.4
NJ	136.8	42.8
NM	137.7	44.5
NY	156.8	23.5
NC	61.0	37.2
ND	66.2	54.6
OH	108.1	32.3
OK	79.6	19.4
OR	96.5	90.9
PA	101.0	52.8
RI	121.3	62.7
SC	69.5	0.6
SD	69.5	65.0
TN	59.9	100.0
TX	90.0	3.8
UT	80.0	81.9
VT	154.1	0.0
VA	77.0	67.8
WA	105.1	99.8
WV	75.8	30.4
WI	85.9	31.8
WY	82.5	0.6

Practice Strategies: A Business Guide for Behavioral Health Care Providers. October, 1997, "Supply and demand in the therapy market," by Gayle Tuttle, p. 6. (*Practice Strategies*™ is published by the American Association of Marriage and Family Therapists. This table is used with permission.)

FIGURE 8.1 Percent of Clinicians per 100,000 Population and Managed Care Medicaid by State (1997)

unique gifts and expertise. Seek out alliances with your colleagues that facilitate working smarter by sharing the time, tasks, and costs of strategic marketing. Creativity will be stimulated as you dialogue and share outreach ideas. Form a supportive professional community to empower confronting these challenges.

Current Marketplace

The *Family Therapy News* (April 1997) in an article "How MFTs Compare to Other Disciplines" (pp. 16, 17, and 26) presented data about clinically trained mental health personnel in the United States. From the largest number to the least, along with the percentage in private practice, the breakdown for the included professional group is as follows:

Type	*Number*	*Percent in Private Practice*
Psychosocial rehabilitation	100,000 (1996)	Not available
Social workers	94,396 (1996)	28
Psychologists	69,817 (1995)	53
Counselors	61,100 (1996)	43
Marriage and family therapists	46,227 (1995)	65
Psychiatrists	33,486 (1995)	46
School psychologists	21,693 (1993)	6
Psychiatric nurses	6,800 (1995)	25

Data are not available for complementary healthcare professionals other than licensed acupuncturists which has 10,000. One might surmise, however, that most complementary therapists would be in private practice. These data represent a large number of mental health professionals who may need skill-building services, products, and resources to assist them in nurturing and growing their practices. Psychologists, marriage and family therapists, psychiatrists, and counselors have the largest numbers in private practice.

Future Marketplace

With supply and demand issues at the forefront for mental health professionals (and perhaps supply and demand issues are beginning to appear as issues for the complementary healthcare providers), the numbers in training are important. The following figures (*Family Therapy News*, April 1997, p. 26) indicate trainees in the various mental health professions (1995 figures):

Type	*Number*
Counseling	30,000
Marriage and family therapy	6,000/7,000
Psychiatric nursing	2,000
Psychiatry	6,000/7,000
Psychology	18,000
Psychosocial rehabilitation (not available)	
School psychology (not available)	
Social work	30,000
Complementary healthcare modalities (not available)	

Graduate schools continue to turn out large numbers of those seeking to enter private practice as well as clinic and hospital based positions. Those entering, particularly if they want to develop a private practice, present a group in need of skill development and business acumen. This is a niche market possibility for the experienced clinician who wishes to network more deeply in her or his professional affiliation as well as to share her or his expertise and wisdom.

More states are licensing and credentialing mental health practitioners and complementary care providers. Contact graduate schools, including schools of massage, acupuncture, and so on, in your area for a mailing list of recent graduates. Contact licensing boards for those licensed within the past two or three years. When marketing to graduate students and/or recent graduates wanting to develop a private practice, you could offer classes in areas such as practice development, management, and marketing. You might also provide supervision of therapy for those preparing to seek licensure.

Another approach is to develop and create continuing education events on basic skills:

- Opening your first office—what's needed?
- Record keeping 101.

- Liability insurance, legal and ethical issues for the beginning practitioner.
- Supervision group for those in practice less than five years.

The Needs of Mental Healthcare Practitioners

Needs are still being shaped by the economy and the paradigm shift in healthcare. In the community mental health field, managed care Medicaid and privatization are making great incursions into funding of public mental health programs. New models are being created, and the field has not as yet stabilized. Stress levels are high; outsourcing and downsizing are occurring often.

Some insurers are beginning to add acupuncturists, massage therapists, and chiropractors to their panels.

In the complementary healthcare field, some insurers are beginning to add acupuncturists, massage therapists, and chiropractors to their panels. This could be a growth area. It is wisdom and good business sense, therefore, to include these professionals within your networking and outreach programs.

Managed care and health maintenance organizations have introduced a night-sea change for the mental health private practitioner. Those therapists whose client base was dependent on insurance company referrals—third-party payments—have seen that base all but evaporate in most states and regions. (If you are in a state that now has a low percentage of citizens in managed care or health maintenance organizations, begin preparing now for their expansion; probabilities are high that further incursions will happen.) Most of us know therapists who are part of the one out of five leaving the field and/or are retiring.

Therapists are going into businesses of bread baking, restauranting, personal/business coaching, bed and breakfasting, humorist, vocational/career counseling, case management, and mediation. Even though therapists have left the field, they most often remain in people-oriented work. In an article focusing on therapists changing careers, Edward Zuckerman, Ph.D., a psychologist who has transitioned into a writer and book editor, says the following (*Family Therapy News*, January/February 1998):

> I don't do therapy anymore, so I don't call myself a therapist, but I can't stop being a psychologist. Like other psychologists, I acquired a worldview that I take with me wherever I go; it is at the core of my being. A bird is a bird no matter where it flies. (p. 26)

Five reasons are noted for therapists transitioning to other careers:

1. Fees are sliding.
2. Incomes are lower.
3. Work weeks are shorter.
4. Interventions are briefer.
5. Third-party payments are smaller.

This information points to a basic need of private practitioners who want to remain in business. That primary necessity is to increase income base to the level that meets their lifestyle. This bottom line amount is different for everyone and correlates with how one defines success for oneself. Your task is to figure that out for yourself and then consider the options and suggestions presented here for creating that wider income base.

This is an area where one's values enter the equation. One grassroots organization in Massachusetts comprises a highly diverse group of therapists who share a common value in simpler living, sustainability, support of and cooperation with one another, the building of a mutual referral system, and accessible mental health services for everyone. They have named themselves the Guild for Financially Accessible Practitioners (see Resources—Organizations).

This is an area where one's values enter the equation.

Some practitioners are relocating to states with more favorable ratios of therapists per 100,000 people. Integrate your values with business acumen either to create or join with the type of networks most reflective of you.

Some practitioners are relocating to states with more favorable ratios of therapists per 100,000 people.

To increase your income base, you need to accomplish the following:

- Learn practice management skills, including ongoing evaluation of the practice.
- Master marketing—the ability to network and to develop outreach materials that address the needs.
- Have a degree of comfort with becoming visible within your therapeutic community and your locale. If you are not already doing so, we encourage you to volunteer within your professional group and join at least one community organization that connects you to referral bases. For example, we are members of the local clergy association and invite them to meet once a year in our offices. We have

also served on boards and committees related to our professional groups. These opportunities raise visibility and provide opportunities for keeping in touch with issues within the professional group and the local community. This knowledge will enable you to develop relevant products and services. Each is also a supportive environment for which there is no price tag. Each is also a referral resource.

- Develop and/or value public speaking capacity/potential.
- Enhance creativity—work smartly and innovatively.
- Take responsibility for your practice.
- Revision your practice—it is best to not have all your eggs in the one basket of the therapy room but to have a diversified income stream.
- Maintain ongoing personal and professional development.
- Keep up with "what's hot" (currently: aging issues of the boomers) as well as "what just keeps on keeping on" (communication skills).

Most of these areas provide opportunities for workshops and seminars for mental health practitioners. If you can, offer continuing education units while earning continuing education units as the presenter. As you become proficient in the preceding areas you can develop skills and abilities that transform successes and failures into products or services for your professional community.

Needs of the Community Mental Health System

Levine and Perkins' book *Principles of Community Psychology: Perspective and Applications* (1997) provides an excellent discussion of this model. Emerging in the mid-1960s during a time of national political and social turmoil, the community mental health/community psychology movement desired to expand greater social justice for the mental health field. The goal and ideal was to relocate the mentally ill from institutionalized settings to the local community. The Community Mental Health Centers Act passed in 1963 and 750 community mental health centers (CMHCs) were founded (one-half the number envisioned).

Deinstitutionalization has birthed new underserved populations and, in urban areas, a ghettoizing and criminalization of the homeless, poor, sick, and mentally ill. Challenges in treating the chronically mentally ill continue. For the community mental health model to work, cooperation among all local institutions, including mental health professionals, is essential. This presents opportunities for private practitioners who are skilled in forming dialogue groups and in teaching or training organizational conflict resolution, mediation, and communication skills.

For the community mental health model to work, cooperation among all local institutions, including mental health professionals, is essential.

In 1992, approximately 227,900 adult mental patients were in publicly funded hospitals. However, during any given year, there may be 3.7 million mentally related hospital episodes (not including children). A large number of these hospitalizations are thought by those in the community psychology modality to be more related to problems in living than to mental disorders.

These figures are indicative of community mental health interests in the social aspects of well-being and stress-related mental illnesses. Resilience in coping with life's difficulties is a major social issue. These areas provide clues for programming and marketing to mental health professionals and complementary healthcare professionals. Development of workshops/seminars related to stress reduction and enhanced resilience can present many opportunities for working with professionals and the community at large.

From Competition to Cooper-tition

In the paradigm of disciplinary professionalism, therapists in private practice and the multiple therapy disciplines were essentially competitors. That paradigm was based on limits rather than on potential, creativity, and the envisioning of expanding venues for your services. It was a replication of the general "moats around the castle" mentality of graduate school programs. In the "civic professionalism" model—a systemic model based on cooperation, collegiality, and bridge building—you should envision the relationship networks you are building as those of mutual support and reciprocity. Envision relationships of an ever-growing complexity that enable development of new outreach services and products, often in collaboration with other mental health/complementary healthcare professionals.

When a crisis is facing a community, such as the one mental health professionals are encountering, survival does not go to the strongest, but to those who are most fit (professionals who are resilient, creative, innovative, and connective). This means creating a more complex system or pattern of interactions rather than withdrawing and/or competitively attempting to take out the competition. These latter styles often lead to burnout and despair. We believe in expanding options and taking different paths—even multiple paths—when your current direction neither moves you toward your goals nor the production of necessary income.

Use your information gathering to interview all mental health professionals with whom you come in contact.

Use your information gathering to interview all mental health professionals with whom you come in contact. Ask them about the population they serve, products and programs they offer, networks they have within their professional group, and within the community. Focus on how you might align and work together on specific projects. Invite them to visit your office and, if they extend an invitation, visit their site. Include their services in your Resource Referral Directory and share these services with the wider community. As you expand your circle, you will meet other like-minded professionals who are open to entering into professional networking relationships. Go with these.

Your Background in the Caregiving Professions

Review your family genogram asking the following questions about your background:

- How many family members were related to the caregiving professions?
- Their gender?
- How many years were they involved in the profession?
- What types of professional crises did or are they experiencing?
- How appreciative of diversity was/is your family?
- How are/were people welcomed into the family?
- What degree of openness/closedness is expressed?
- How resilient was your family in the midst of work stress and crisis (i.e., job loss, transitioning to new career, change in lifestyle)?
- What are major features of their response to stress/crisis?

- Other questions and/or observations about your family of origin?
- What is the impact of the preceding on your professional style?

Review your therapeutic school family-of-origin. Reflect on your graduate school experiences. Ask any of the preceding questions that may be relevant, as well as the following:

- What did you learn and/or hear about your particular school of thought from your supervisors, mentors, professors?
- What where their biases and prejudices? Were these discussed?
- What did you hear and/or learn about other therapy schools?
- Was there cross-pollination of ideas and techniques between the various schools?
- What is your current comfort level with practitioners of other styles of therapy?
- Which, if any, do you have respect for? Which do you have the most questions about?
- Which would you like to learn more about?
- Did you take any business classes in college? Was therapeutic work ever discussed from the business perspective? Was income ever discussed in your classes?
- What is the current environment like in your graduate school program? Is the program growing? Have there been changes? What do you hear from the school? From former professors?
- What is the impact of this on you and on your practice style? On your belief system about yourself as a private practitioner?
- What did you need to adapt, relearn, learn, and/or change to transition into the paradigm we are suggesting?
- What do you celebrate and affirm about your training? About your practice?
- Other questions?

Exploring these questions about your family-of-origin and your therapy school family-of-origin prepares you to move more intentionally and connectedly within mental health and complementary healthcare perspectives.

Transferable Skills

As therapists, we know that building relationships with our clients has a great deal to do with the therapy/counseling outcome. The same is true as you consider other mental health practitioners as an area for marketing your practice. Be patient. After you have done your planning and started to put it into practice, allow the time for relationship and trust to develop. Monitor your progress and be attuned to the feedback you receive. Allow for adaptability and redirection; allow for redoubling your efforts at some point in the cycle (see Chapter 1, Figure 1.3). Plan for such phases in your schedule.

Monitor your progress and be attuned to the feedback you receive.

Throw a wide net when inviting cooperation. The final number will likely be smaller than the number of initial responses. From that smaller group, you will find those who are like-minded, share compatible values, and are committed to being responsible for their part in agreed on, shared tasks and outreach activities. If reciprocity and mutuality are not present, it won't work. Be clear about expectations.

The skills, abilities, and unique gifts you bring to your practice are the same ones you bring to your outreach efforts. Many of your colleagues are confronted with and suffering from the same social challenges you are. Each of us in the healthcare sector needs support during this tumultuous time. Just as attorneys have a proverb saying: "An attorney who has him- or herself for a client is a fool," so trying to be one's own therapist/counselor is also foolish. Your colleagues may be experiencing needs where you have transferable skills:

- Crisis and/or trauma.
- Life transitions—job changes, injuries and illness, separations and divorces, grief and loss.
- Clinical issues such as depression, anxiety, and personality disorders.
- Couple and family concerns.
- Need of resourcing/referring to specialists.
- Interviewing, evaluation, assessment and intervention models.
- Knowledge of practice development and management.

- Professional identity issues.
- Refashioning of a practice or expansion of a skill base—vocational and/or career coaching/consulting/counseling.

Demythologizing the professions enables us to see our colleagues and ourselves as human beings in search of meaning and purpose in life. When changed circumstances challenge meaning and purpose, we are in as much need, and need as much compassion, as our clients.

What Makes You Special?

As an empathic man or woman, your knowledge base about the human condition and what is helpful to others makes you unique among the professions. These qualities are just as needed among peers as among other members of the population. Enlarge your purview to include this marketing venue for your services and product development.

Specific niche area possibilities are:

- Supervising newcomers in the field and facilitating peer supervision. Consider becoming a certified supervisor in your professional group.
- Writing for publication as a way of attaining visibility and expertise in certain areas (e.g., practice development, enhancing creativity, career transitions, sharing your clinical passions).
- Becoming trained in instruments such as the Myers-Briggs, and their uses for couples, career assessment, writing, research.
- Working cooperatively with complementary caregivers.
- Working cooperatively with community mental health professionals.
- Developing and presenting life-skills programs. Offer workshops to community mental health programs as well as the community at large. There is great interest in the following: marriage, giving birth, parenting, divorce, living with chronic illness, sexuality.
- Developing community education materials on mental resilience and mental illness. (If materials are available, you can use and adapt them to your locale and to your style.)
- Developing a woman-to-woman or man-to-man professional practices group with your female or male colleagues. Include

complementary caregivers (massage therapists, chiropractic, acupuncture, etc.) and market your services to other men's and women's professional groups such as attorneys, physicians, and business professionals.

- Creating training programs for mental health professionals who want to add public speaking to their skills.
- Team-building for mental health professionals.
- Developing presentations and workshops around national observance days such as National Depression Screening Day, National Anxiety Depression Screening Day, Eating Disorders Day, Mental Health Week, and Mental Health Month.

Use your creativity along with your knowledge of your local community and region.

Use your creativity along with your knowledge of your local community and region.

As a mental health professional, you bring a wealth of knowledge and ability to whatever pursuit you choose. Use your knowledge and ability to benefit both your colleagues and yourself.

Engaging the Marketplace

Making a Match

Here are some possibilities as you begin connecting with the mental health and complementary care practitioners in your area:

- Arrange a series of open houses directed toward the mental health groups you want to network and perhaps team with.
- Volunteer with your particular mental health profession.
- Have a booth at annual conferences of your organization as well as at as many of the other groups of mental health and complementary care professionals as you can afford (invite other practitioners to attend with you and share the booth cost).
- Volunteer and/or attend meetings of a professional group in your community.

When participating in these activities, note the practitioners with whom you feel resonance and share similar values. Talk with them about mental health and/or complementary care practice, ask questions about interests, abilities, and their vision for practice. Follow up with these contacts and explore potentials for cooperation and collegiality around professional support and codevelopment of products and services. Allow for the relationship building and process time essential for success. Be patient. Simultaneously, keep your focus on the goals of building a sustainable and thriving practice by attending to your marketing plan.

Follow up with these contacts and explore potentials for cooperation and collegiality around professional support and codevelopment of products and services.

Marketing Plan

In your marketing plan, sort out those products/services that you want to develop and offer as an individual and those you would like to develop with other professionals. Since the latter is a mutual activity, arrange a meeting with like-minded practitioners. Invite attendees to come with their ideas, share them, and see what arises from the mix. Having a combination of individual products and services along with team offerings is a nice combination. Each activity enriches the whole.

The following tools are helpful for developing each service/product, whether a solo or a team effort. The examples are for marketing to mental health professionals and can be adapted for complementary healthcare providers as well as community mental health practitioners.

Figure 8.2 shows a mindmap for developing a mailing/contact list for caregivers. Figure 8.3 is a goal sheet for developing a Depression Day Screening Team.

Services and Products

In addition to the following, several possibilities have been mentioned in prior sections. Review them to stimulate your own ideas:

- *Education/Information.* There remains a tremendous need for education and information about mental illness. Clients have many concerns about medications and often are ill informed about them as well as the common experiences of depression and/or anxiety. Mental and emotional problems continue to be perceived as something shameful. Estimates are that 40 million adult Americans will have a mental disorder at some point in their life. Hope and wellness need to be shared with our communities. Create a panel with other practitioners and present a program at local organizations, schools, and so on.

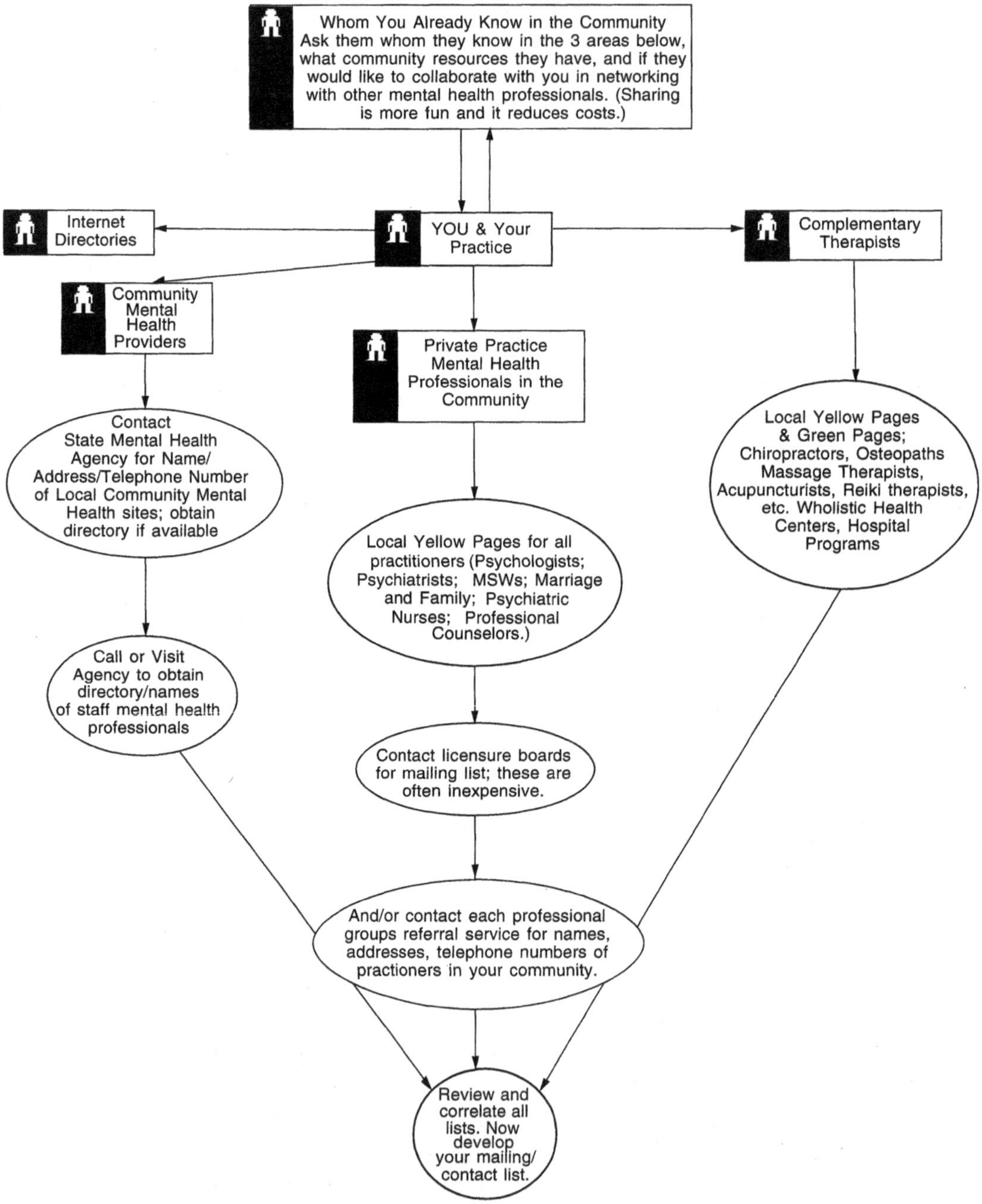

FIGURE 8.2 Mental Health and Complementary Therapists Networking Mindmap

Today's Date: 12/31/98

Step	Task	Target Completion Date
!	My Goal is: Participate in Depression Screening Day with a team of at least four; one being a complementary therapist and one being from the community mental health center.	Target Completion Date: June 30, 1999
1	Gather directories: yellow pages, green pages, referral system of professional organizations	Target Completion Date: February 5, 1999
2	Create Mailing list	Target Completion Date: February 15, 1999
3	Write introductory letter with invitation to Spring open house (4/30/98) and to share in Autumn Depression Screening Day. Depression Screening Day materials to be at Open House for review. Develop brochure, create resource directory sheet & mail-back card. Print # needed.	Target Completion Date: February 30, 1999
4	Address envelopes and mail to selected mailing list.	Target Completion Date: March 15, 1999
5	Call those who have responded, Confirming open house date & inviting them to bring their brochures, etc. for a networking table.	Target Completion Date: April 5, 1999
6	Prepare materials for open house; sign-in sheets, your marketing materials, creative name tags, arrange for refreshments, flowers, networking table, display of Depression Screening Day materials, tv & video machine for viewing video, etc	Target Completion Date: April 28, 1999
7	At Open House, speak to your desire to co-sponsor Depression Screening Day with a diverse group. If those who sign up on the "interest sheet" are not as inclusive as you wish, target those representative of what you envision and invite their specific	Target Completion Date: April 30, 1999
8	Gather those interested and set a follow-up discussion-planning meeting to consider location for screening day, scheduling the day, costs, etc.	Target Completion Date: May 15, 1999
9	Location decided, confirmed, and materials ordered for Autumn event. September review meeting scheduled.	Target Completion Date: June 30, 1999

FIGURE 8.3 Sample Goal Setting Worksheet for Mental Health and Complementary Health Care Professionals

- *Visibility and Networking.* Team with other community mental health organizations around shared events during National Alcohol and Drug Addiction Recovery Month (or similar event).

Obtain kits and consider these options:

- *Library.* Ask your library to set up a table with selected titles on alcohol and drug addiction. The library could also sponsor a workshop or presentation open to the community. (Whenever you participate, have your outreach materials available.) Videos are available for showing, followed by discussion and questions and answers.

Provide materials to local churches, synagogues, and mosques.

- *Literature.* Provide materials to local churches, synagogues, and mosques. Offer yourself and/or panel as a speaker to religious groups about addictions or other important community interests related to mental well-being.
- *Community Organizations.* Develop a Parent-Teacher Organization (PTO) program. Offer to speak and bring fact sheets related to children and adolescents.
- *Public Relations Releases.* Inform local news organs about National Alcohol and Drug Addiction Recovery Month.
- *Media Contacts.* Volunteer to be interviewed by the media.
- *Joining with Complementary Therapists.* Offer continuing education for mental health practitioners (and a community education event) about the various modalities; for example, "Counseling Therapies and Complementary Paths to Well-Being." A program like this could also be offered to cable television or local radio.
- *Educational Videos.* An example is the Bill Moyers series *Healing and the Mind.* Sponsor and facilitate a 5-week educational series in conjunction with colleagues and complementary healthcare providers. Transcripts are available. The videos may be purchased through Ambrose Video Publishing, 1290 Avenue of the Americas #2245, New York 10104; or call (800) 843-0048.
- *Entrepreneurial "Hot Issues."* For example, develop a niche working with older adults and/or their families. One-fourth of the American population is over 50.

Important concerns are sandwich generation issues, grandparents raising grandchildren, elderly depression, and suicide. The top six aging concerns are (clues here for developing products or services): (1) appearance, (2) sexuality, (3) disease, (4) memory loss, (5) income-producing ability, and (6) access to quality healthcare.

Practitioners will be treating increasing numbers of the aging, including the aging who are in caregiving roles. There is increased potential of numbers suffering from overstress, depression, anxiety, substance abuse, and so on. Consider completing a certificate program in geriatric psychology or take continuing education classes on aging issues. Network with other professionals in the classes to develop programs. An excellent book for an alternative, empowering view of the aging process is *From Age-ing to Sage-Ing: A Profound New Vision of Growing Older*, by Zalman Shachter-Shaloma and Ronald S. Miller (Warner, 1995). For more information contact:

Practitioners will be treating increasing numbers of the aging, including the aging who are in caregiving roles.

The Spiritual Eldering Institute
7318 Germantown Avenue
Philadelphia, PA 19119
(888) 353-7464

The United Nations has designated 1999 International Year of Older Persons. The theme is "Toward a Society for All Ages"—obtain study materials and resources from the UN (see Resources).

- *Web Site and Chat Room.* Join together with colleagues to develop a web site; offer your products and services on the web. Have a chat room and share the schedule of "being there" to discuss pertinent issues.
- *Certified Care Manager.* Investigate expanding your services to elderly and the sandwich generation by becoming a certified care manager. For information:

  National Academy of Certified Care Managers
  P.O. Box 666
  244 Upton Road
  Colchester, CT 06415-0666
  (800) 962-2260

- *Teams, Couples, and Marital.* Train in use of a tool or instrument, which can be a mechanism for marketing such as Myers-Briggs, Enneagram. Offer as a 2- or 3-session enrichment program for mental health and other teams and couples.

Use your resourcefulness and initiative to create programs for the mental health and complementary healthcare professional.

Outreach Vehicles

The bottom line here is to develop outreach materials directed to needs rather than to intellect. Advertisements can be quite inexpensive when placed in newsletters of professional groups. When you team up with colleagues and share the cost, your overhead expenses are reduced, which means more money in your pocket.

Advertisements in Professional Newsletters

When marketing to mental health and complementary care practitioners, visibility is as important a component to your success as it is to any other professional group. Reflect on the many possibilities you can create to enhance your visibility.

Mental Health/Complementary Care Practitioner Referral Resource Directory Worksheet

This is an important tool for networking and developing mutual referral systems. When you do a new mailing, always include a Resource Directory Worksheet to be returned to you. Have copies available at your booth when you are at conferences, and so on.

Letters

Figures 8.4 and 8.5 show sample letters for communicating with your colleagues. Adapt them to your style and locale.

Alpha Centre

6 Pleasant Street   Suite 214   Malden MA 02148   617-322-3051

Our mission is to be a professional resource in support of the health and well-being of
- The whole person
- Families
- Businesses, institutions, and
- Municipalities

in the service of creating caring community

Our services include psychoeducational workshops on:

GROWING YOUR PRACTICE

MARKETING TO NICHE GROUPS:
- RELIGIOUS GROUPS
- PHYSICIANS
- ATTORNEYS
- EDUCATORS
- COMPLEMENTARY THERAPISTS
- MENTAL HEALTH PROFESSIONALS

RELATING TO THE MEDIA

PEER SUPERVISION GROUPS

MARKETING SUPPORT GROUPS

INDIVIDUAL CONSULTING & COACHING

CAREER/VOCATIONAL COUNSELING

CONTINUING EDUCATION EVENTS

Dear ___________ :

We know you provide a tremendous amount of services with limited resources. We at the Alpha Centre believe that community mental health providers are primary resources for supporting and enhancing the well-being of our community. We are writing to get to know you better.

As a service to our clients, we keep a Resource Directory of every mental health and complementary service in our area. this helps with referral to others to fill the needs of those we work with. Please fill in the information requested and return it to us in the self-addressed-return envelope. As a thank-you we are enclosing a copy of one of our informational newsletters we offer to colleagues and clients free of charge.

The Alpha Centre for Counseling and Mediation serves the mental health needs of the citizens of Malden, Medford, Melrose and surrounding communities. Together, we have many years of counseling experience. We offer services to individuals, couples, children, family, and groups to heal and enhance relationships. We believe this trickles down to improve the emotional and mental well-being of our community.

A brochure describing services is enclosed with the Resource Directory Worksheet. PLEASE, complete it and return to us.

If you are interested in any in-service psychoeducational programs on the topics to the left, please contact us. In addition we will work with you on topics related to your particular interests and needs.

As mental health professionals we are sensitive to and respectful of diversity, multicultural and confidentiality issues. We are interested in meeting and discussing with you ways in which we might serve as resources to you and your colleagues. We look forward to meeting you and working together on behalf of our shared community life.

We will call within the next week to arrange an interview date to follow up on the Directory Worksheet.

Sincerely,

FIGURE 8.4 Introductory Letter to Community Mental Health Center

Dear _________ :

We certainly feel the challenges and concerns around maintaining a private practice and know that many of our colleagues share similar feelings. On September 10, 1999, we will begin offering the following year-long group for mental health professionals. Our hope is that this supportive group offering will assist everyone in nurturing the self and their private practice.

The group focus includes issues of practice development and strategic marketing. We cover the following topics:

August 7 - The Self of the Therapist:
September 10 - Why You Chose a Mental Health Professional and How That Can Guide You in Your Professional Development
October 8 - Collaboration with Colleagues for Strategic Practice Building
November 12 - Innovative Interventions for Difficult Cases
December 10 - Becoming a "Co-Creator" - Discovering the Artist Within
January 9 - "Thinking Outside the Box"
February 13 - Developing Your Sense of Humor
March 13 - Contemporary Ethical Issues and Dilemmas
April 11 - Personal and Professional Resilience
May 14 - The Professional's Stress Reduction Toolkit

13.5 CEUs applied for. Group size limited to 12.
Cost: $20 per group session; commitment to all sessions necessary.
Group will meet 2:00-4:00 pm on scheduled dates.

Enclosed is a copy of our brochure and a Resource Directory Information Sheet. Please complete the form and return to us. We use it to make referrals for clients with members of the community.

If you have any questions, please contact us at 781.322.3051. We hope you will join us for the group meetings.

Sincerely,

FIGURE 8.5 Sample Letter Announcing New Group

Mail-Back Card

Communication is two-way. When you do a mailing, always invite a response. Including a mail-back or fax-back card is one way to do this. Another is to request a telephone call if the recipient of your mailings has questions or comments.

Newsletter

Developing a newsletter for the particular professional groups with which you want to network is another helpful way to gain visibility, name recognition, and grow your practice. Depending on the time you have, it can be monthly or quarterly. Focus your feature article on what will be informative for the reader. In the examples following, Figure 8.6 is directed toward mental health professionals; Figure 8.7 is directed toward complementary healthcare professionals. With the aid of desktop publishing as well as preprinted newsletters, creating newsletter mailings has become greatly simplified both as to time and to cost. Be creative. (If you team up, sharing the cost reduces overhead.)

Telephone Script

Because the schedules of mental health professionals range from regular to irregular, it is a good idea to first call and arrange a time for a telephone conversation. When you have your telephone appointment, the following script is a guide for directing the conversation; adapt it to your style and location. Be open and listen well. Keep the call focused. Follow up with a note. A sample telephone script is shown on pages 272–273.

To Do List

Having several methods to maintain accountability with your marketing and outreach vehicles will help you accomplish your strategic marketing plan. A simple To Do list will facilitate such accountability and focusing your time and budgeting. Create a to do list for any marketing project you develop. A sample list appears on page 274.

Alpha Centre

June 1998
Volume 1, Issue 1

Inside this Issue

Alpha Centre
6 Pleasant St. #214
Malden MA 02146
781.322.5051

SERVING THE NEEDS OF ELDERS

This information is offered as a practice development resource for mental health and complementary healthcare professionals. For more copies, articles on other aspects of practice development, and information about consultation and coaching, contact The Alpha Centre @ 781.322.3051

Substance abuse in the elderly is largely undiagnosed and undertreated. Statistics are startling. Consider the following:

• 3 million seniors over 60 are alcoholic.

• the highest rate of alcoholism in America is found in widowers 75+ years of age.

• those over 65 account for 25% of all prescriptions while comprising only 11% of the population.

• 90% use non-prescription drugs

Those most at risk share the following in common:

• loss of loved ones

• identity concerns.

• struggled with substance abuse in younger years.

• have medical conditions that involve pain and loss of sleep.

• are emotionally ill -- depression,

Schizophrenia, etc.

• confusion about taking their prescription medications.

Symptoms to look for: sleeplessness, memory loss, chronic health complaints, shaky hands, poor hygiene and unkempt appearance, important tasks left undone, crying, defensiveness about drinking and/or drugs.

Studies have shown that although seniors may at first feel a great deal of shame about their addiction they can be very responsive to treatment and do well in treatment programs geared toward their age group.

Because of ageism and misconceptions about the aging process, physicians rarely diagnose alcoholism or substance abuse. One study found that 80% of physicians diagnosed it as depression; another found that only 1% considered it even when encountering the symptoms.

(Adapted from "Addiction in the Golden Years", by Jan Marie Werblin, October 1998, pp. 25-28, Professional Counselor Resources

Resources

Alcoholism in the Elderly: Diagnosis, Treatment, and Prevention. Department of Geriatric Health, American Medical Association, 515 N. State Street, Chicago, IL 60610. Telephone: 312-464-5085.

"How to Talk to an Older Person Who Has a Problem with Alcohol or Medications". Obtain from the Hazelden Web site at http://www.hazelden.org or call 1-800-I-DO CARE.

Assessment Tool

Michigan Alcoholism Screening Test - Geriatric Version (MAST-G)

Developed to evaluate alcoholism in older clients, the following 24 questions could be useful for other age groups. 5

FIGURE 8.6 Newsletter for Mental Health Professionals

or more "yes" answers may be indicative of alcohol problems.

1. After drinking have you ever noticed an increase in your heart rate or beating in your chest? Yes______ No______

2. When talking with others, do you ever underestimate how much you actually drink? Yes____ No_____

3. Does alcohol make you sleepy so that you often fall asleep in your chair? Yes_______ No______

4. After a few drinks, have you sometimes not eaten or been able to skip a meal because you didn't feel hungry? Yes____ No_____

5. Does having a few drinks help decrease your shakiness or tremors? Yes_____ No_______

6. Does alcohol sometimes make it hard for you to remember parts of the day or night? Yes___No___

7. Do you have rules for yourself that you won't drink before a certain time of the day? Yes___No__

8. Have you lost interest in hobbies or activities that you used to enjoy? Yes____ No____

9. When you wake up in the morning, do you ever have trouble remembering part of the night before? Yes__ No ___

10. Does having drink help you sleep? Yes ___ No___

11. Do you hide your alcohol bottles from family members? Yes ___ No___

12. After a social gathering, have you ever felt embarrassed because you drank too much? Yes ___ No___

13. Have you ever been concerned that drinking might be harmful to your health? Yes___No___

14. Do you like to end an evening with a nightcap? Yes___ No___

15. Did you find your drinking increased after someone close to you died? Yes___ No___

16. In general, would you prefer to have a few drinks at home rather than go out to social events? Yes___ No___

17. Are you drinking more now than in the past? Yes___ No____

18. Do you usually take a drink to relax or calm your nerves? Yes ____ No____

19. Do you drink to take your mind off your problems? Yes ___ No___

20. Have you ever increased your drinking after experiencing loss in your life? Yes___ No___

21. Do you sometimes drive when you have had too much to drink? Yes___ No____

22. Has a doctor or nurse ever said they were worried or concerned about your drinking? Yes___ No___

23. Have you ever made rules to manage your drinking? Yes___ No____

24. When you feel lonely does having a drink help? Yes___ No___

For more information about the test contact: Frederic Blow, PhD, University of Michigan Alcohol Research Center, and 400 E. Eisenhower Pkwy. Suite A, Ann Arbor, MI 48104. Telephone: 734-998-7952. (Professional Counselor, p. 48, October 1998).

Marketing Tips

Marketing Tip 1: Obtain one of the free brochures in resources and mail it with a cover letter, the assessment tool, and your brochure to physicians in your community inviting their response.

Marketing Tip 2: Offer a community education presentation/workshop at the local library on the topic. Develop a panel to present: Therapist, substance abuse expert, physician and/or nurse, acupuncturist, etc. Have marketing materials available.

Continuing Education Events

"The Self of the Therapist:

Linda and Jean will be co-facilitating a monthly group for practitioners September May. We look forward to a diverse group of 12 participants and will focus on the following September 10: "Why I choose to be a practitioner. "

October 8: "Collaboration with colleagues & strategic practice building"

November 12: "Innovative interventions for difficult cases"

December 10: "Discovering the artist within"

January 9: "Outside the box" thinking"

February 13: "Developing My Sense of Humor"

March 13: "Ethical issues and dilemmas"

April 11: "Personal and Professional Resilience"

May 14: "My stress reduction toolkit"

13.5 CEUs applied for. Cost: $20 per group session; commitment to all sessions required. Group will meet 2:00-4:00 PM on scheduled dates.

Come Join Us! Our motto?

"To make our calendar, it must be fun!"

Web Site of Interest

Women's Health Information Center/U.S. Public Health Service: http: www.4woman.gov. This site has links to all federal agencies and publications dealing with women's health, including numerous government screened private organizations. Telephone: 1-800-994-9662. Fact sheets, brochures and other printed materials.

2

FIGURE 8.6 *(Continued)*

Alpha Centre

Alpha Centre

June 1998
Volume 1, Issue 1

Inside this Issue

1 Alpha Centre

1 Complementary Therapists

2 Marketing Tips

2 Educational Opportunities....... And more

Self-Direction – Never be bullied into silence. Never allow yourself to be a

Victim. Accept no one's definition of your life; rather, define it yourself.

Harvey Fierstein

Hope – To hope means to be ready at every moment for that which is not yet born, and

Yet not become desperate if there is no birth in our lifetime.

Erich Fromm

Alpha Centre
6 Pleasant St. #214
Malden MA 02146
781.322.5051

A Professional Community Resource

Linda L Lawless LMFT LMHC CGP
Jean Wright, DMin., LMFT LMHC

The Alpha Centre mission is to be a professional resource in support of the health and well being of
• the whole person
• families
• business, institutions, and municipalities
in the service of creating caring community

What is a caring community?
Our vision of a caring community is one in which individuals, families, businesses, institutions and municipalities put the welfare of the person before profit or power. In order for this to become a reality, everyone involved must embrace this primary value. We can only begin one step at a time and we have begun with ourselves. We invite others to engage in a dialogue about how we can all put people first.

An example at the Alpha Centre is our referral service. When someone calls looking for a mental health professional, if we cannot provide the services needed we use a therapist finder to locate someone who can be of help at the closest geographic location possible. We invite other health professionals to use our referral service. From the 978 or 781 area code, call 1-800-THERAPIST. From other area codes call 781.322.3051. Leave your name, number, and the reason for your call and someone will return your call promptly.

We use a wholistic approach to wellness and invite dialogue with all human healthcare professionals to expand our understanding of how we can help those in need. If you are a professional who is interested in networking, please contact us @ 781.322.3051.

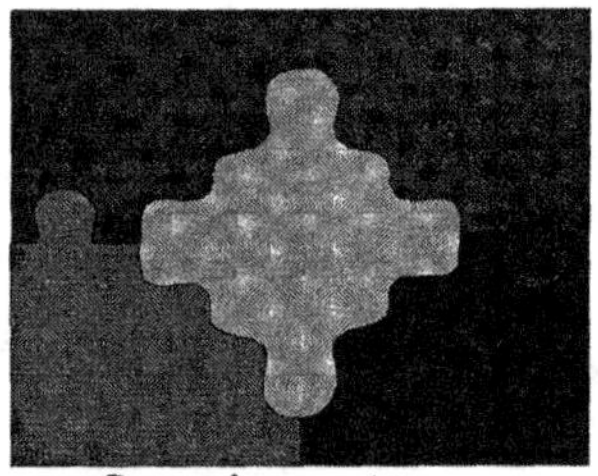

Complementary Therapists

Exciting News

Boston Regional Medical Center, Stoneham, MA, recently announced that its Complementary Medicine Program is now a training site for masters of acupuncture degree students at the New England School of Acupuncture (NESA), located in Watertown, MA. The teaching affiliation between NESA and BRMC is one of the first clinical affiliations in the United States between a hospital and an Oriental medicine college and the first in New England.

Harvard-Vanguard HMO (Health Maintenance Organization) recently announced that access to alternative therapies such as chiropractic, massage and acupuncture are now available at the Cambridge, Burlington, Quincy and

1

FIGURE 8.7 Newsletter for Complementary Health Professionals

June 1998

Kenmore offices; such services will be expanding to other locations in 1999. They want to improve communication between the traditional and alternative caregivers.

Did You Know?

Over 30 medical school now offer courses in alternative medicine including Harvard, Columbia Stanford and Georgetown.

A 1993 Harvard medical school study found that 2/3 of Americans had relied on some form of alternative medicine in the previous year.

A September 1998, survey of 1,000 Americans by the Stanford University School of Medicine found that 69 % had used alternative therapy in the previous year - the majority for preventive reasons and usually while also seeing a medical doctor.

Talking to the Media

Now that a public dialogue/debate is happening between practitioners of complementary health care modalities and the traditional modalities, you may receive inquiries from reporters requesting an interview. Be prepared and consider the following guidelines:

1. **Know** the message you want to communicate - have specific information rather than generalities. Prior to the interview, choose points you want to make. Write them down; refer to them.
2. **Sound bites** are the way. Have some good quotable information. For instance such as in the above "Exciting News".
3. **Reflect upon from the reporter's perspective**. He/she may know little about alternative therapies. Educate them about your own. Offer other resources such as websites, people, book, etc. (Be a resource to the media.)
4. **Who is the audience?** Respond in a way that the average women/man "on the street" will understand. If it's televised, image and voice are important. If it's radio, voice is important. If it's to be written, quotability and information is important. Seek advice and practice. (Viewers/Hearers/-readers are potential clients.)
5. **Remain calm and in control**. Stay focused on your message and points. Ask for clarification about questions if unsure. Correct any misstatements by the reporter. Breathe!
6. **It's an opportunity - take advantage. Be Yourself.** After the reporter uses the piece, send a thank-you note. You'll be remembered for the next time.

Marketing Tip 1:
Use the opportunity of the current national discussion about complementary health care to call your community newspaper and offer an op-ed piece or column about your specialty and the field. You may also do this for the local cable channel. These folk are often receptive.

Marketing Tip 2:
Offer a community education presentation-workshop at the local library or other public site. Develop a panel to present: Therapist, physician and/or nurse, acupuncturist, etc. Announce in the newspaper. Have marketing materials available.

Upcoming Event

Whole Health Expo
October 13-15, 1999
Bay Road Center

The Alpha Centre will have a booth. If you are interested in sharing space with us, please call 781.322.3051. Share the fun! Cut the cost!

The Expo is a great time and place for networking and learning about what is on the horizon regarding paradigms and products.

Web Sites of Interest

1. National Women's Health Information Center/U.S. Public Health Service: http: www.4woman.gov. This site has links to all federal agencies and publications dealing with women's health, including numerous government screened private organizations. Telephone: 1-800-994-9662. Fact sheets, brochures and other printed materials.

2. Deepak Chopra Websites:
http://www.chopra.com
www.randomhouse.com/site/chopra

3.www.americanwholehealth.com/awh/htm [Physician Supervised Alternative Medicine]

4.www.mindbodyspirit.org/welcome.htm

Upcoming Continuing Education Events

"The Self of the Therapist:
Linda and Jean will be co-facilitating a monthly group for practitioners September-May. We look forward to a diverse group of 12 participants and will focus on the following:

September 10: Why I choose to be a practitioner.
October 8: Collaboration with colleagues on strategic practice building
November 12: Innovative interventions for difficult cases
December 10: Becoming a "co-creator"- discovering the artist within
January 9: " Outside the box" thinking
February 13: Developing My Sense of Humor
March 13: Ethical issues and dilemmas
April 11: Personal and Professional Resilience
May 14: My stress reduction toolkit

13.5 CEUs applied for.
Cost: $20 per group session; commitment to all sessions required.
Group will meet 2:00-4:00 PM on scheduled dates.
For more information: 781-322-3051

Come Join Us! Our motto,
"To make our calendar, it must be fun!"

Some copy in this newsletter was provided by First Draft, a desktop publication resource. 1-800-878-5331

2

FIGURE 8.7 *(Continued)*

Telephone Script

Preparing. The mental health professional and/or complementary healthcare professional you are calling has received your letter and brochures in advance.

- Have a copy of the materials before you.
- Review your family-of-origin genogram and your therapy family-of-origin as it relates to marketing to the mental healthcare community. Be in a place of comfort with the relationships.
- Call or schedule the telephone appointment at a time when you are most likely to feel refreshed and confident.
- Be prepared to not make contact on the first call; do not hesitate to call back.
- Be prepared to focus and take charge of the call. Remember that your agenda is to begin building relationships.
- Take a deep breath and place the call.

Connecting:

- You may get an answering machine and/or an answering service. Either way, identify yourself and your practice and ask to speak with Mr./Mrs./Dr. "Smith." Share that you are responding to his or her request for information if the mail-back card has been returned. If not, say that you are calling to discuss your mailing with him or her. Identify yourself as a colleague. If you know a person in common, identify that person as having recommended "Smith" to you. You will most likely receive a high priority. If he or she is not available, ask that your call be returned, leaving your telephone number with times you may be reached. If you do not receive a return call within a day or two, do not hesitate to call again. Create a follow-up note to call again.
- You reach the mental health/complementary care professional. Have your script at hand and follow it. Keep your text to one page and remember that the call is about building a relationship. In your first paragraph, you begin building a relationship. Introduce yourself and your business; mention that you are a licensed mental health professional.

  This is ______, of ______. I'm a licensed ______ and have been located in (name of community) since ______. (If you know someone who knows the therapist, mention the person's name and your relationship to him or her at this time. Let this person also know that you will be talking soon with the person.) Share a positive bit of input, for example, "Barbara/Paul shared with me that you have a deep interest in supporting children/families where divorce is being experienced. I share that interest and am trained in family and divorce mediation," and so on.

Presentation. This comprises the second paragraph and contains your reason for calling:

> "Did you receive the letter and brochure I mailed on ______? Do you have questions, comments about it? "

Share why you want to network with your colleagues (your particular specialties that correlate with the colleague's areas of expertise) and that you believe that you share mutual interests, which can benefit you both.

- Ask how long have they been in practice. How did they become interested in the work? Be interested and keep your questions specific to the topic.
- Ask whether they collaborate with mental health professionals in the community. If so, ask about the collaboration and mention any common ground you share. You may also base comments on your mission statement. Invite the therapist's ideas about common ground (e.g., families of divorce) and include comments about your training and experience in the field. Share that you respect confidentiality issues.

This will aid in building the bridges of trust and openness. Ask if there are regular meetings of therapists in the community to which you might be invited. If so, to whom would you speak about the possibility of attending? Offer yourself as a speaker on a topic of interest to them. Can he or she be helpful or is there another contact? If so, who is that person?

Close. The third paragraph brings closure to the telephone meeting. If all has gone well and you feel that there is a like-minded interest, invite the educator to lunch or ask for an appointment to meet and further discuss how you might assist one another. Make appropriate thank-yous and close with a "looking forward to meeting you in person" statement.

Affirming. Give yourself a pat on the back! You're on your way to building a network with colleagues in your local community.

Completing. Follow up the telephone call with a note stating that you appreciate the time taken and that you look forward to the possibility of working together around your common interests in the future. If you have scheduled a luncheon meeting and/or appointment to meet, mention it.

To Do List

- Gather Yellow Pages and appropriate directories and select out those practitioners who are compatible with your location by [date].
- Look in the Yellow Pages for your psychological association referral service and obtain names/addresses/telephone numbers of psychologists in your area by [date].
- Check applicable web sites of therapists in your locality by [date].
- Check sources, previously noted, for complementary healthcare professionals by [date].
- List the practitioners you already know; obtain addresses and telephone numbers (date to call their office for possible referrals to other therapists).
- List names of friends, family, and colleagues who might be able to supply names of therapists (date to call them).
- Call [date].
- Prepare mailing to attorneys by [date].
- Develop brochure by [date].
- Write cover letters by [date].
- Develop and write enclosures by [date].
- Develop and write newsletter by [date].
- Mail packet by [date].
- Note calendar calling date [date].
- Review telephone script and practice aloud by [date].
- Integrate all dates with your Goals Plan.
- Mail telephone follow-up note by [date], for example:

  Dear ______:

  It was a pleasure to learn of your interest and experience in the ______ arena. I enjoyed speaking with you and appreciated your time taken. As we both work with ______ in often-difficult situations, it is good to have a resource in the field of addictions counseling for referrals. I look forward to future contact with you. Please do not hesitate to contact me if you have further questions.

Summary

Consider marketing products and services to your colleagues and peers as you would any other professional group. To have a successful, thriving practice, mental health practitioners need just as many business tools as other businesspeople. They also need support to evoke, develop, and mature the business side of their professional life. Confront issues related to this reality within yourself and use that as additional ground for deepening your relationships to your own professional group as well as others within the circle of health, healing, and well-being. Again, stresses shared are lessened! Successes shared are multiplied!

Resources

Internet

Aging Resources

Better Health web site—www.betterhealth.com

American Geriatrics Society—www.americangeriatrics.org/

American Society on Aging—www.asaging.org/

Gerontological Society of America—www.geron.org/

U.S. Administration on Aging—www.aoa.dhhs.gov/aoa/pages/info.html

Social Security Administration—www.ssa.gov/

Medicare Information—www.Medicare.gov/

American Association for Geriatric Psychiatry—www.aagpgpa.org/

Alzheimer's Association—www.alz.org/

National Family Caregivers Association—www.nfcacares.org/

Family Caregiver Alliance—www.caregiver.org/

Alternative and Complementary Medicine

Alternative and Complementary Therapies Conferences—www.alternativemed.com

American Academy of Medical Acupuncture—www.medicalacupuncture.org (800) 521-2262

Association for Integrative Medicine—www.integrativemedicine.org/

Deepak Chopra Web-sites—www.chopra.com

East/West Institute of Alternative Medicine—www.eastwestinstitute.com

Expressive Therapies and Arts Medicine—www.expressivetherapy.org/
Herbal Medicine Practitioners—visit Dr. Andrew Weil's web site—www.drweil.com
Mind, Body, Spirit—www.mindbodyspirit.org/welcome.htm
Physician Supervised Alternative Medicine—www.americanwholehealth.com/
Study Web–Health and Nutrition—www.studyweb.com/health/nutrit/
Whole Life Expo—www.wholelifeexpos.com

Anxiety Disorders
Anxiety Disorders Association of America—www.adaa.org

Assessment Resources
Psychological Assessment Resources, Inc.—www.parinc.com

Biofeedback
EEG Spectrum—www.eegspectrum.com
Stens Corporation—www.stens-biofeedback.com

Child and Adolescent (see Resources in Chapter 6)
Youth Change—www.youthchg.com

Computer Classes
Ziff-David University (online computer classes)—www.zdu.com

Jungian Seminars
www.jungianseminars.org

Psycho-Legal Associates
http://members.aol.com/psylegal/www/info.html

Psychology/Mental Health/Managed Care
American Mental Health Counselors Association—www.amhca.org
Alternatives to Managed Care Page—www.hmopage.org
American Mental Health Alliance—www.mental-health-coop.com
American Psychological Association—www.apa.org/
Association for Advancement of Behavior Therapy—www.aabt.org/aabt

Guide to Internet Therapists and Counselors—www.metanoia.org/
Psychology and Technology—www.psychotechnology.com

Psychological Modalities
American Association of Marriage and Family Therapists—www.aamft.org/
Beck Institute—www.beckinstitute.org
Christian Association for Psychological Studies—www.caps.net
EMDR Training—www.emdr.com
Imago Therapy—www.imagotherapy.com
International Society for the Study of Dissociation—www.issd.org/
Milton H. Erickson Foundation— www.erickson-foundation.org/

Traditional Medicine
American Medical Association—www.ama-assn.org/
Harvard Health Publications—www.harvardhealthpubs.org
Human Brain Project—www.scripps.edu/
New England Journal of Medicine—www.nejm.org/content/index.asp
On-line Health and Medical Journals—www.healthfinder.gov/

Women's Health/Mental Health
The Renfrew Center—www.renfrew.org
National Women's Health Information Center—www.4woman.gov
(800) 994-9662

U.S. Government
List of U.S. federal government agencies—www.lib.lsu.edu/gov/fedgov.html

National Screening Days (a sampling)

National Anxiety Disorders Screening Day
c/o Freedom from Fear
308 Seaview Avenue
Staten Island, NY 10305

National Community Mental Healthcare Council—to obtain Mental Health Month Kit
12300 Twinbrook Parkway, Suite 320
Rockville, MD 20852
(301) 984-6200

National Depression Screening Day
Douglas G. Jacobs, MD, Director
One Washington Street, Suite 304
Wellesley, MA 02181
(617) 239-0071
Fax: (617) 431-7447

Journals/Newsletters/Magazines (a sampling)

Alternative Medicine Magazine
21½ Main Street
Tiburon, CA 94920
(415) 789-8700
Fax: (415) 789-9138

Common Boundary: Exploring Psychology, Spirituality, and Creativity
4905 Del Ray Avenue
Bethesda, MD 20814
(301) 652-9495
e-mail: connect@commonboundary.org
www.commonboundary.org

Community Mental Health Journal
NCMHC
12300 Twinbrook Parkway, Suite 320
Rockville, MD 20852

Harvard Women's Health Watch
Harvard Medical School Health Publications Group
164 Longwood Avenue
Boston, MA 02115

***Health Wisdom for Women* (Dr. Christian Northrup's Newsletter)**
Phillips Publishing
7811 Montrose Road
Potomac, MD 20854
(800) 804-0935

Holistic Health Guide for New England
Spirit of Change
P.O. Box 410
Grafton, MA 01519
(508) 650-1471
Fax: (508) 839-1173
e-mail: sosie@gateway.net

InService: Continuing Education Opportunities for Counseling and Therapy Professionals
3800 Quentin Street
Denver, CO 80239
(888) 690-5214
Fax: (303) 574-9049

Managed Care Strategies
13901 U.S. Highway 1, Suite 5
Juno Beach, FL 33408
(561) 624-1155
Fax: (561) 624-6006

Mind & Body Health Newsletter
The Center for Health Sciences
c/o ISHK Book Service
P.O. Box 381069
Cambridge, MA 02238-1069
(800) 222-4745

Open Minds: The Behavioral Health Industry Analyst
10 York Street, Suite 200
Gettysburg, PA 17325-2301
(717) 334-1329
Fax: (717) 334-0538
e-mail: openminds@openminds.com
www.openminds.com

Practice Strategies: A Business Guide for Behavioral Healthcare Providers
Gayle Tuttle & Associates, Inc.
442½ East Main Street, Suite 2
Clayton, NC 27520
(919) 552-0637
Fax: (919) 553-4584

Psychology and Health Update
P.O. Box 469103
Escondido, CA 92046-9103

Psychotherapy Finances
13901 U.S. Highway 1, Suite 5
Juno Beach, FL 33408
(561) 624-1155
Fax: (561) 624-6006
www.psyfin.com

Medical Libraries (geared to laypeople)

Center for Medical Consumers
237 Thompson Street
New York, NY 10012
(212) 674-7105

Planetree Health Resource Center
2040 Webster Street
San Francisco, CA 94115
(415) 923-3680

National Organization for Rare Diseases (NORD)
P.O. Box 8923
New Fairfield, CT 06812
(203) 746-6518

***Grateful Med* (an online resource for accessing medical databases)**
Available for $29.95 from:
U.S. Commerce Department
National Technical Information Service
Springfield, VA 22161
(703) 487-4650

Medical Research Firms That Will Research Databases for You

The Health Resource
564 Locust Street
Conway, AR 72032
(501) 329-5272
($275 for research on cancer; $175 for other topics)

Planetree Health Resource Center
2040 Webster Street
San Francisco, CA 94115
(415) 923-3680
($100 per report)

Schine On-Line
39 Brenton Avenue
Providence, RI 02906
($189 for cancer research; $100 for other illnesses)

Organizations

Academy for Guided Imagery
P.O. Box 2070
Mill Valley, CA 94942
(800) 726-2070

Academy of Family Mediators
5 Militia Drive
Lexington, MA 02421
(781) 674-2664
Fax: (781) 674-2690
e-mail: AFMoffice@mediators.org
www.mediators.org/

American Association of Sex Educators, Counselors and Therapists (ASSECT)
P.O. Box 238
Mt. Vernon, IA 52314-0238
(319) 895-8407
Fax: (319) 895-6203
e-mail: AASECT@worldnet.att.net

American Group Psychotherapy Association
Dept. 1, 25 East 21st Street
6th Floor
New York, NY 10010
(212) 477-2677
Fax: (212) 979-6627

American Massage Therapy Association
820 Davis Street, Suite 100
Evanston, IL 60201
(847) 864-0723
Fax: (847) 864-1178
e-mail: infor@inet.amtamassage.org
www.amtamassage.org

American Mental Health Alliance of New England
P.O. Box 1036
Cambridge, MA 02140-0009
(617) 576-9900

American Polarity Therapy Association
2888 Bluff Street, Suite 149
Boulder, CO 80301
(800) 359-5620
Fax: (303) 545-2161
e-mail: SATVAH@aolcom
www.polaritytherapy.org

American Society on Aging
833 Market Street, Suite 511
San Francisco, CA 94102-1824
(800) 537-9728
Fax: (415) 974-0300
www.asaging.org

American WholeHealth, Inc.
Corporate Headquarters
1150 Sunset Hills Road
Reston, VA 20190
(703) 437-6336
e-mail: Questions@AWHINC.com

Anxiety Disorders Association of America (ADAA)
11900 Parklawn Drive, Suite 100
Rockville, MD 20852
(301) 231-9350
Fax: (301) 231-7392
e-mail: anxdis@aol.com
www.adaa.org

Association for Psychological Type
9140 Ward Parkway, Suite 200
Kansas City, MO 64114
(816) 444-3500
Fax: (816) 444-0330
email: training@aptcentral.org
www.aptcentral.org

Association of Private Practice Therapists (APPT)
P.O. Box 241621
Omaha, NE 68124-5621
(402) 333-1197
Fax: (402) 333-1658

Bureau of Essential Ethics Education
P.O. Box 80208
R.S.M., CA 92688-0208
e-mail: ethicsusa@home.com
www.ethicsusa.com/

Coalition for Marriage, Family and Couples Education LLC
5310 Belt Road NW
Washington, DC 20015-1961
(202) 362-3332
Fax: (202) 362-0973
e-mail: CMFCE@smarmarriages.com
www.smartmarriages.com

Expressive Therapy Concepts
P.O. Box 1
Mont Clare, PA 19453
www.expressivetherapy.org/

Guild for Financially Accessible Practitioners Network (GAP-NET)
P.O. Box 162
Newton, MA 02159
(617) 244-5542

Image Paths, Inc.
P.O. Box 5714
Cleveland, OH 44101-0714
(800) 800-8661

Institute for Trauma and Loss in Children
900 Cook Road
Grosse Pointe Woods, MI 48236
(313) 885-0390
Fax: (313) 885-1861

National Academy of Certified Care Managers
3389 Sheridan Street, #170
Hollywood, FL 33021
(800) 962-2260

National Alliance for the Mentally Ill
200 North Glebe Road, Suite 1015
Arlington, VA 22203-3457
(800) 950-6264
www.nami.org

National Association of Alcoholism and Drug Abuse Counselors
1911 North Fort Myer Drive, Suite 900
Arlington, VA 22209
(800) 548-0497
Fax: (800) 377-1136 or (703) 741-7698
www.naadac.org

National Career Development Association
4700 Reed Road, Suite M
Columbus, OH 43220

National Clearinghouse for Alcohol and Drug Information
P.O. Box 2345
Rockville, MD 20852
(800) 729-6686
www.health.org/

National Mental Health Association
1021 Prince Street
Alexandria, VA 22314-2971
(800) 969-6642
www.nmha.org

National Mental Health Consumers
Self-Help Clearinghouse
1211 Chestnut Street, 11th Floor
Philadelphia, PA 19107
(800) 553-4539

National Mental Health Services
Knowledge Exchange Network (KEN)
P.O. Box 42490
Washington, DC 20015
(800) 789-2647
Fax: (301) 984-8796
www.mentalhealth.org
(A wealth of information, including substance abuse)

New England Holistic Counselors Association
P.O. Box 525
Portsmouth, RI 02871
(401) 683-1723

New England School of Acupuncture
34 Chestnut Street
Watertown, MA 02472
(617) 926-4271
www.nesa.edu

Society for Light Treatment and Biological Rhythms, Inc.
10200 West 44th Avenue, Suite 304
Wheat Ridge, CO 80033-2840
(303) 422-7905
Fax: (303) 422-8894

The Spiritual Eldering Institute
7318 Germantown Avenue
Philadelphia, PA 19119
(888) 353-7464

Whole Person Associates, Inc.
210 West Michigan
Duluth, MN 55802-1908
(218) 727-0500

Recommended Reading

Aldridge, D. (1993, Fall). Is there evidence for spiritual healing? *Advances: The Journal of Mind-Body Health*, 9(4), 4–21.

Amber, R. (1983). *Color therapy: Healing with color.* New York: Aurora Press.

Ambrose, J. (1997, April). How MFTs compare to other disciplines. *Family Therapy News, 28*(2), 16–17, 26.

Barnett, R.A. (1997). *Tonics: More than 100 recipes that improve the body and the mind.* New York: Harper Perennial.

Bassman, L. (1998). *The whole mind: The definitive guide to complementary treatments for mind, mood, and emotion.* Novato, CA: New World Library.

Benson, H. (1997). *Timeless healing: The power and biology of belief.* New York: Simon & Schuster.

Benson, H., & Klipper, M.Z. (1976). *The relaxation response.* New York: Avon Books.

Benson, H., & Proctor, W. (1985). *Beyond the relaxation response.* New York: Berkley.

Boorstein, S. (1996). *Transpersonal psychotherapy* (2nd ed.). Albany: State University of New York Press.

Borysenko, J. (1988). *Minding the body, mending the mind.* New York: Bantam Books.

Capuzzi, D., & Gross, D.R. (1999). *Counseling and psychotherapy: Theories and interventions* (2nd ed.). Upper Saddle River, NJ: Merrill.

Carlin, J. (1992, July/August). Whatever happened to community mental health: Steering through the storm. *The Family Therapy Networker, 16*(4), 24–25, 59.

Carolson, R., & Shield, B. (Eds.). (1989). *Healers on healing*. Los Angeles: Jeremy P. Tarcher.

Chodorow, J. (1991). *Dance therapy and depth psychology: The moving imagination*. New York: Routledge.

Chödrön, P. (1997). *When things fall apart: Heart advice for difficult times*. Boston: Shambhala.

Chopra, D. (1993). *Ageless body, timeless mind: The quantum alternative to growing old*. New York: Harmony Books.

Cornish, E. (Ed.). (1996). *Exploring your future: Living, learning, and working in the information age*. Bethesda, MD: World Future Society.

Dossey, L. (1996). *Healing words: The power of prayer and the practice of medicine*. San Francisco: HarperCollins.

Dubovsky, S.L. (1997). *Mind-body deceptions: The psychosomatics of every day life*. New York: Norton.

Farhi, D. (1996). *The breathing book*. New York: Henry Holt.

Foss, L., & Rothenberg, K. (1987). *The second medical revolution: From biomedicine to infomedicine*. Boston: New Science Library.

Gawain, S. (1982). *Creative visualization*. New York: Bantam Books.

Gordon, J. (1996). *Manifesto for a new medicine: Your guide to healing partnerships and the wise use of alternative therapies*. Boston: Addison-Wesley.

Gottschalk O.K. (1989). *The encyclopedia of alternative healthcare*. New York: Pocket Books.

Hackney, H.L., & Cormier, L.S. (1993). *The professional counselor: A process guide to helping* (3rd ed.). Boston: Allyn & Bacon.

Hendricks, G. (1991). *RADIANCE: Breathwork, movement, and body-centered psychotherapy*. Berkeley, CA: Wingvow Press.

Hendricks, G. (1995). *Conscious breathing: Breathwork for health, stress release and personal mastery*. New York: Bantam Books.

Hendricks, G., & Hendricks, K. (1993). *At the speed of life: A new approach to personal change through body-centered therapy*. New York: Bantam Books.

Hunt, M. (1994). *The story of psychology*. New York: Anchor Books.

Jennings, S. (1987). *Drama therapy: Theory and practice for teachers and clinicians*. Cambridge, MA: Brookline Books.

Kettering Review. (1996, Summer). Community [Special issue]. *Kettering Review*.

Konner, M. (1993). *Medicine at the crossroads: The crisis in healthcare*. New York: Pantheon Books.

Levine, M., & Perkins, D.V. (1997). *Principles of community psychology: Perspective and applications* (2nd ed.). New York & Oxford: Oxford University Press.

Loman, S. (Ed.). (1992). *The body-mind connection in human movement analysis*. Keene, NH: Antioch University.

Lowman, R.L., & Resnick, R.J. (Eds.). (1994). *The mental health professional's guide to managed care*. Washington, DC: American Psychological Association.

Lusk, J.T. (1992–1993). *30 scripts for relaxation imagery and inner healing* (Vols. 1 and 2). Duluth, MN: Whole Person Associates.

McKay, M., & Paleg, K. (Eds.). (1992). *Focal group psychotherapy*. Oakland, CA: New Harbinger.

Micozzi, M.S. (Ed.). (1996). *Fundamentals of complementary and alternative medicine*. New York: Churchill-Livingstone.

Miller, J.L. (1998, December). On the web. *Professional Counselor*, 18–19.

Mindell, E. (1998). *Earl Mindell's supplement bible*. New York: Simon & Schuster.

Morrison, M.R., & Stamps, R.F. (1998). *DSM-IV internet companion: A complete guide to over 1500 web sites offering information on mental illness, keyed to DSM-IV*. New York: Norton.

Mowrey, D.B. (1993). *Herbal tonic therapies: Information on how more than 60 healing herbs can help your heart, your immune system, your nerves and your whole body*. New York: Wings Books.

Northrup, C. (1998). *Women's bodies, women's wisdom: Creating physical and emotional health and healing*. New York: Bantam Books.

O'Donohue, W., & Krasner, L. (Eds.). (1995). Handbook of psychological skills training. *Clinical Techniques and Applications*. Boston: Allyn & Bacon.

Opler, L.A., & Bialkowski, C. (1996). *Prozac and other psychiatric drugs: Everything you need to know*. New York: Pocket Books.

Payne, H. (Ed.). (1993). *Handbook of inquiry in the arts therapies: One river, many currents*. London: Jessica Kingsley.

Provider profiles. (1998, August). *Practice Strategies*, p. 7.

Ramacus, T. "Alternative Therapies Reference Library." Site guide at: http://altmedicine.abort.com.

Rossi, E.L. (1993). *The psychobiology of mind-body healing: New concepts of therapeutic hypnosis*. New York: Norton.

Sachs, J. (1994). *The healing power of sex*. Englewood Cliffs, NJ: Prentice Hall.

Schulz, M.L. (1998). Awakening intuition: Using your mind-body network for insight and healing. New York: Harmony Books.

Seaburn, D.B., Lorenz, A., Gawinski, B.A., Gunn, W., & Mauksch, L.B. (1996). *Models of collaboration: A guide for mental health professionals working with healthcare practitioners*. New York: Basic Books.

Shachter-Shaloma, Z., & Miller, R.S. (1995). *From age-ing to sage-ing: A profound new vision of growing older*. New York: Warner.

Sobel, D.S., & Ornstein, R. (1996). *The healthy mind, healthy body handbook*. Los Altos, CA: DRx.

Szasz, T.S. (1961). *The myth of mental illness*. New York: Dell.

Tuttle, G.M. (1997, October). "Supply and demand in the therapy market." *Practice Strategies: A Business Guide for Behavioral Health Care Providers*, pp. 1, 6.

Tuttle, G.M., & Woods, D.R. (1997). *The managed care answer book for mental health professionals.* Bristol, PA: Brunner/Mazel.

Weil, A. (1990). *Natural health, natural medicine.* Boston: Houghton Mifflin.

Weil, A. (1995). *Spontaneous healing.* New York: Knopf.

Weil, A. (1997). *Eight weeks to optimum health.* New York: Knopf.

Wilson, E.O. (1998). *Consilience: The unity of knowledge.* New York: Knopf.

Woody, R.H. (1997). *Legally safe mental health practice: Psychological questions and answers.* Madison, CT: Psychosocial Press.

Wylie, M.S. (1992, July/August). Whatever happened to community mental health: Revising the dream? *Family Therapy Networker, 16*(4), 10–23.

Wylie, M.S. (1998, January/February). Breaking free: Career change as a liberating experience. *Family Therapy Networker, 22*(1), 25–33.

9

The Community Connection

The community is a complex marketplace. This chapter explores the wellness and prevention services that the community can use. However, it does not address the one million plus untreated mentally ill who are homeless or residing in the community because of deinstitutionalization. Serving this very ill population requires a network of outreach services that was not put into place when state hospitals were downsized. As a result, it is difficult to work with this group as a whole. We continue, however, to be proactive in supporting our communities in their struggles to deal with people who clearly need many kinds of care. Before you reach out to your community, you must ensure that your outreach efforts are meant to improve the common good. Len Duhl, who helped create the World Health Organization's Healthy Cities Program, lists six characteristics of a healthy city, which conversely sound reminiscent of a healthy person:

1. Healthy cities have a sense of history to which their citizens relate and upon which their commonly held values are grounded.
2. Healthy cities are multidimensional and have a complex and interactive economy.
3. Healthy cities strive for decentralization of power and citizen participation in making decisions about policy.
4. Healthy cities' leaders focus on the whole of the city and can visualize both parts and "wholes" simultaneously.
5. Healthy cities can adapt to change, cope with breakdown, repair themselves, and learn from their own experience and that of other cities.
6. Healthy cities support and maintain their infrastructure (*Inner Edge,* August/September 1998).

Healthy cities are much like healthy people. Unless you firmly believe what you have to offer adds value in creating and maintaining the health of your community and are willing to put yourself, your services, and products up for public scrutiny, this marketplace is not for you. Psychotherapists usually practice in their offices, protected by confidentiality, receiving referrals from known sources. To reach out to the community at large through public speaking and workshops, written pieces, and other forms of public relations requires full visibility. You need to share personal information about your strengths and weaknesses to strike a personal chord in your audience and make a connection that they trust.

Before you reach out to the community, you need to decide which one you are going to focus on—the one you live in or the one you practice in (if they are different). When you connect with your community of choice, you will be receiving referrals that pay in multiple ways (insurance, private pay, cash, credit card). Be prepared to screen for those you prefer to work with and be prepared to bill in the preferred model. If you want to accept credit cards, consult with your professional association about those arrangements.

You need to decide which one you are going to focus on—the one you live in or the one you practice in.

History of Your Community

Get to know your community. What is its history? What memorable events helped shape its character? What commercial developments created its commerce? Recent demographics show that in the United States, with a population of 52 million people, 29.5 percent of people ages 15 to 54 and 14.7 percent of of the general population have mental or addictive disorders and receive services for their problems. Your community will have its own mental health demographics. Go to the municipal offices and seek out any community studies that have been done by the local government or local hospitals or mental health agencies. Use the Internet to gather more information about your community. There are many resources on the Internet to help you. These are the national gateway sites you can begin with:

Use the Internet to gather more information about your community.

- City Link www.banzai.neosoft.com/citylink/ma.html
- City Net www.city.net/countries/united_states/massachusetts/
- Yahoo! Government www.yahoo.com/Government/

Date: ______________________________ New: _____ Revision: _____

Name: ______________________________

Address: ______________________________

Organization: ______________________________

Telephone(s): ______________________________

Fax: ______________ E-mail: ______________ Website: ______________

Office Hours: ______________ Handicapped Accessible: Y ______ N ______

Parking Available: Y _____ N ______ Public Transportation Available: Y _____ N _____

Languages Spoken: ______________________________

Type of Population you Serve: ______________ Sliding Scale Fee: Y _____ N _____

Insurance Accepted: Y ____ N ____ Types: ______________

Licenses/Certifications Held: ______________________________

Specialities Offered: ______________________________

Professional Affiliations: ______________________________

What else is important that would help with a potential referral? ______________

____

____

Thank you for completing this Resource Directory Form.

Mail to:
Alpha Centre
6 Pleasant Street Suite 214
Malden, MA 02148
or Fax to 781.322.3051

If you have any questions, please call: 781-322-3051
Linda Lawless, MA, LMFT/LMHC; Jean Wright, DMin, LMFT/LMHC

Source: Adapted from L. Lawless *Therapy Inc.* (New York: John Wiley, 1997). Reprinted with permission.

FIGURE 9.1 Community Resource Directory Worksheet

The federal government has sites on the Internet that include the United States Government Printing Office and THOMAS, which provides the full text of U.S. legislation and the *Congressional Record* and links to other sites. The U.S. General Services Administration Federal Telecommunications Service Office of Network Applications hosts the Government Information Exchange, a directory of government Internet resources.

Gather information from the schools about student needs and talk to local community leaders about the town's history of needs and services. Some town libraries keep a room that is dedicated to local history and local authors. The Practice Resource Directory presented in *Therapy Inc.* (Lawless, 1997) ". . . serves a twofold purpose. First it is your insurance that you know about all the resources in your area. Second, it is your way of letting others know who you are . . ." Use the Practice Resource Directory worksheet, adapted for your community, to begin to get the lay of the mental health land in your community (Figure 9.1).

Categorize businesses by the kinds of services they provide (e.g., mental health, educational). In any given category, list what is provided and look for what is missing. Look at the big picture of your community and then focus on its mental health and wellness needs.

Categorize businesses by the kinds of services they provide.

Your Community Values and Beliefs

What is your commitment to the community? Do not enter this marketplace if you do not plan on being a long-term player. What are your community values and beliefs? If you have difficulty networking and reaching out to the public, this is not the niche for you. This market requires a love of group involvement. A possible mission statement for a mental health professional reaching out to the community is "To help people face new experiences and change in their personal and work lives. To enhance a sense of community, stimulate creative thought, and facilitate discussion and resolution of mental health community problems." Believe that the community will be open to you as you develop your capacity for connectedness and develop the resources you have to offer. It is good to be prepared before you enter this market. The checklist on page 290 will help you determine how well prepared you are for this market.

____ I am able to speak up about issues in a group and share my ideas.

____ I enjoy a healthy dialogue about differing perspectives.

____ I can say "no" to requests for my resources when they would be in excess of my abilities to give.

____ I am in touch with my emotions when I speak, can stop talking when my point has been communicated, and do not harbor ill feelings toward others who were unable to listen or differ in opinion.

____ I am able to stay present in groups, and hear and see what is going on in an objective manner.

____ I do not resort to my "professional expertise" to make a point when I believe I am not being listened to.

____ Under no circumstances, would I abuse the power of my professional standing in the community.

Engaging the Community

After you have an overview of your community, you need to look to your skills and specialties and find what you can offer that will meet your community's needs. There is the specialty approach and the general mental health approach. Look at others in your field as collaborators, not competitors. Any community project is too big for one person. You will all need help. Consider your particular specialties and narrow the parts of the community you can best serve. Remember that "mental health" often carries a stigma. You must be ready, internally and externally, to manage this stigma and reframe mental wellness as a mainstream benefit to individuals and their community. You must be wellness oriented. Nobody wants to attend a workshop on suffering. For personal inspiration, we have enjoyed the readings we have found in *The Inner Edge: A Resource for Enlightened Business Practice,* contact: (800)899-1712. They offer articles on business and community that inspire creative change.

Consider your particular specialties and narrow the parts of the community you can best serve.

Where do you start in connecting with the community? The National Issues Forum model helps you organize a forum/study circle around a specific community issue. You bring together 12 people and meet in a community building, or your office. There are two leaders, the convenor and the moderator, who bring the group to their task. The convenor puts the meeting together, and the moderator facilitates the discussion. Start small. The goal of the group is to bring citizens together to work through community problems and reach solutions. The convenor clarifies the unifying purpose of the group and networks with others that have self-interest in addressing the identified problem. The National Issues Forum has created materials you can use for many community issues, contact: (800)433-7834. These include moderator guides, videotapes, and direction in creating and running an issue forum.

General Calendar Approach

If creating a focus group does not appeal to you, you can target individuals, businesses, and the local government by offering a particular resource or specialty, or you can reach out with written publications during seasonal and special events. Allow the event to stimulate your ideas. For example, during Human Resources Month, contact a local EAP and ask how you can help make their life easier. For regional specific events, check your state's home page and your local community's calendar for their special events. They may have an annual fair or city celebration. Any special city, or calendar, event creates a natural outreach topic (e.g., "Christmas—Holiday Blues: Dealing with seasonal depression"). You need to be in touch with the community's "agenda" so you can be part of its future. The national months in the following list remain constant, the weeks, and days change. To know what week and day they fall on and to find graphic arts you can use for your outreach pieces, subscribe to Dynamic Graphics, a copyright-free graphic service we have found helpful for our desktop publishing. For sponsorship information, use your local library's resource librarian to help you track them down. We have listed a few mental health oriented sponsors to give you an idea of who generates these special months, weeks, and days (see May). For more detailed information, use the "Health Observances and Recognition Day Calendar." Contact: Society for Healthcare Strategy and Market Development (800) 242-2626 or *Chase's Calendar of Events—The Day-to-Day Directory to Special Days, Weeks, and Months* (312) 540-4500.

If creating a focus group does not appeal to you, you can target individuals, businesses, and the local government by offering a particular resource or specialty, or you can reach out with written publications during seasonal and special events.

January

- New Year's Day
- National Eye Health Month
- Human Resources Month
- National Clean-Off-Your-Desk Day
- Make Your Dreams Come True Day
- World Religion Day
- National School Nurse Day
- Veterans Day

February

- Eating Disorders Awareness & Prevention Week EDAP (206) 382-3587
- Relationship Skills (Valentines Day)
- American Heart Month
- National Blah Buster Month
- Be an Encourager Day
- Groundhog Day
- Torture Abolition Day
- National Have a Heart Day
- Presidents' Day

March

- Brain Awareness Week—Charles A. Dana Foundation www.dana.org/brainweek
- National Women's History Month
- Foot Health Month
- I Want You to Be Happy Day
- TV Turn Off Day
- National Procrastination Week
- Panic Day

True Confessions Day
St. Patrick's Day
American Chocolate Week
Memory Day
National Goof Off Day
Make Up Your Own Holiday Day
Passover

April

Easter
Earth Day
Keep America Beautiful Month
National Anxiety Month
National Humor Month
Prevention of Animal Cruelty Month
Stress Awareness Month
April Fool's Day
Remembrance Day
Victims of Violence Holy Day
Earth Day
National Honesty Day

May

May Day
Mother's Day
Memorial Day
Be Kind to Animals Week
National Teachers Day
National Nurses Week
Police Week

Breaking Through the Stigma—sponsored by the National Council for Community Behavioral Healthcare. Their packet must be purchased. Contact them at (301) 984-6200

National Mental Health Month (NMHA) (703) 684-7722

Stroke Awareness Month

National Physical Fitness and Sports Month—President's Council on Physical Fitness (202) 690-5179

Better Sleep Month—Better Sleep Council (703) 683-8371

Older Americans Month—U.S. Administration on Aging (202) 401-4541

National Anxiety Disorders Day—Freedom from Fear (718) 351-1717

Children's Mental Health Week—Missouri Statewide Parent Advisory Network (314) 972-0600

Childhood Depression Awareness Day—NMHA (703) 684-7722

National Nursing Home Week—American Health Care Association (202) 842-4444

National Employee Health and Fitness Day—National Association of Governors' Councils of Physical Fitness and Sports (317) 237-5630

June

International Mothers' Peace Day

Teacher "Thank You" Week

National Flag Week

Family History Day

National Forgiveness Day

Adopt a Shelter Cat Month

Flag Day

Father's Day

July

4th of July

Pleasure Week

Freedom Week

National Therapeutic Recreation Week

Anti-Boredom Month

National Purposeful Parenting Month

August

National Alcohol and Drug Addiction Recovery Month. To be a sponsor and receive a kit that includes promotional ideas, press releases, media advisory, radio scripts, and a logo sheet, contact Department of Health and Human Services, Rockville MD (800) 843-4971

First National Alcohol Screening Day (NASD), contact NMISP/NASD (781) 239-0071 www.nmisp.org

National Eye Exam Month

Psychic Week

National Smile Week

National Relaxation Day

Be Kind to Humankind Week

Women's Equality Day

September

Baby Safety Month

National Courtesy Month

Self Improvement Month

Child Accident Prevention Week

Labor Day

Swap Ideas Day

National Chiropractic Week

National Grandparents Day

National Singles Week

Yom Kippur

National Good Neighbor Day

National Alcohol and Drug Addiction Recovery Month

October

- Halloween
- National AIDS Awareness Month
- World Vegetarian Day
- Mental Illness Awareness Week
- Columbus Day
- National Grouch Day
- National Business Women's Week
- Evaluate Your Life Day

November

- Thanksgiving
- Child Safety and Protection Month
- National Epilepsy Awareness Month
- Veterans Day
- National Stop the Violence Day

December

- Universal Human Rights Month
- World AIDS Day
- Chanukah
- Tell Someone They're Doing a Good Job Week
- Bill of Rights Day
- National Whiner's Day
- Kwanzaa

Wellness Oriented Services

As healthcare access becomes more complex and difficult, people are beginning to take more control of their health through education and lifestyle change. Through the Internet, clients can access health information that was never available to them before. They are not only finding resources for their illnesses; they are also trying to prevent illness. Our culture is moving from a model of psychopathology to one of a positive psychology. The National Institute of Mental Health (NIMH) is focusing on psychological strengths and how these "protective factors" can prevent mental illness:

> They catalogued four principle domains of psychological strengths: self/personal; cognitive; biological/temperamental; and occupational/social. They defined seven dimensions of personal resilience: insight; independence; relationships; initiative; creativity; humor; and morality. They defined the hardy personality: as consisting of a sense of commitment, a positive response to challenge, and an internal locus of control. They identified the importance of hopefulness, as opposed to hopelessness. (The Group Circle, February/March 1999)

MCOs are also looking at prevention services to offset clinical utilization of services. We have listed a few of the wellness-oriented approaches you, with your specialized training, can effectively offer as workshops and consultative opportunities for the public.

Life Extension. Our population is getting older and many people are interested in quality of life as they age. *The Longevity Strategy: How to live to 100 using the brain-body connection* (Mahoney & Restak, 1998) is an excellent approach to this issue. It can be used as a model for consultation and psychoeducational programs. It addresses the many things individuals can do to extend their lives and increase their current wellness. Workshops you could develop that relate to this issue are:

Stress management	Humor and longevity
Positive thinking techniques	Mental fitness
Life balance	Safe risk taking
The art of optimism	Active retirement

Healthy change is another issue that informed consumers are seeking.

Change Management. Healthy change is another issue that informed consumers are seeking. There are many approaches to this topic. Some topics are:

- Developing rituals for positive change.
- Lifestyle change and self-management—A how-to model.
- Laughter training.
- Lifetime reading for self-improvement.

Child Protection. Almost all families are concerned about the safety of their children. The Polaroid Corporation and the National Center for Missing and Exploited children have created a program for missing and exploited children. Project KidCare photographs children for free. The picture is placed in a book with vital information that the parent keeps in case the child is ever missing. A free guidebook to hold a Project KidCare event is available from Polaroid at (800) 662-8337. This is the kind of event you can host in your office.

Agencies. A video is available from the California Association of Marriage and Family Therapists (CAMFT) entitled "Shadows to Light," which was produced by California's Attorney General. It portrays educators, doctors, and others discussing their feelings about their roles in protecting children. It is ideal for private and public agencies that deal with victims of child abuse or their abusers. CAMFT can be reached at (619) 292-2638.

Many state and local governments are focusing on parenting programs.

Parenting. Offer free parenting classes. Many state and local governments are focusing on parenting programs. Twenty-five states have adopted parenting programs. This will create a need for in-home psychoeducational resources. Contact state governments, school systems, and local social service agencies to find out what their needs are and what groups they are serving (e.g., the Massachusetts social workers visit expectant teenagers, and in Texas there is a special parent education program for Latinos).

Family Therapy. Strengthening the family is a foundational issue for creating healthy communities. This is being recognized more and more by state agencies. Florida requires marrying or divorcing couples to take family classes and requires a licensed mental health professional or clergy to teach the course. Typical topics for families are:

Premarital testing	Stepparenting
Couples counseling	Divorce recovery
Mediation services	Relationship issues
Parent survival training	Child loss support groups

Many businesses have created training and psychoeducational programs that you can use with confidence in your own practice. Some of them are:

- PREPARE/ENRICH Workshops. Offers training programs to certify you to use their training program and assessment materials. For information contact them at (800) 331-1661 or visit their web site at www.lifeinnovation.com
- Connections—Relationships and Marriage by Charlene R. Kamper. "A program designed for teens to learn and experience the benefits of positive relationships." For a sample lesson call The Dibble Fund at (800) 695-7975.
- Partners—Curriculum for preserving marriages. A project of the American Bar Association's Fund for Justice and Education. They offer a training program that includes a videotape and curriculum manual. Contact them at (630) 455-9192 or order from the American Bar Association, Publication Order (312) 988-5522.
- Stepfamily Association of America. Has training programs, books, tapes, and videos. Order their catalog by calling (800) 735-0329.
- Family Wellness Associates. Offers instructor training in their program. To receive a catalog and information about their training, call (408) 426-5588 or visit their web site at www.familywellness.com
- PAIRS—Practical Application of Intimate Relationship Skills. Offers a certification training to present their marriage programs. Contact them at (954) 431-4540 or visit their web site at www.pairs.com

Certification. Become a Certified Family Life Educator by contacting the National Council on Family Relations. Call (888) 781-9331 or visit their web site at www.ncfr.com.

Publications. Offering free or low-cost publications to your clients and the public is a win-win marketing approach. You can publish your own newsletter or order publications that are already in place. An example is *Marriage Magazine*. You can subscribe to this publication and order past issues for 25 cents to use as giveaways for clients or at public speaking events. For a sample copy, contact them at (800) 627-2424.

The Teacher and Parent Training Catalogue—Childswork Childsplay—lists other publications you can sell or give away. Contact them at (800) 962-1141.

Coaching

Entering the coaching field is an easy transition for mental health professionals.

Entering the coaching field is an easy transition for mental health professionals. Coaching can be done over the telephone, in your office, or out in the field. Clients are business professionals, sales executives, entrepreneurs, lawyers, brokers, and so on. To flourish in this niche, you need to have good communication skills and understand the coaching model. Abraham Maslow spoke about the "unconscious competence" of self-actualizing persons and their capacity to sustain energy and be highly effective in many settings. That is what coaches are about. A coach grounds clients in their core values and beliefs, inspires challenging future scenarios, facilitates optimal choices through visionary plans, and guides the successful enactment of those plans through training, networking, and ongoing coaching. As a coach, you can offer your services to the community.

A resource for this topic is the Hudson Institute at (800) 552-4401, or visit their web site at www.hudsoninstitute.com/coaches.

Specialty-Oriented Services

Sports Psychology

The sports psychology specialty is a growing field. Certification requires a doctorate degree and 400 hours of supervised counseling experience. More information can be obtained from the Association for the Advancement of Applied Sport Psychology (AAASP) (519) 661-4118, University of Western Ontario, London, Ontario. They have a quarterly newsletter that you can order by calling the office of the *Journal of Applied Sport Psychology*, (800) 627-0629.

Trauma Recovery

Trauma is a daily event in most communities, some worse than others. Trauma recovery can mean recovering emotionally from a major medical trauma (e.g., heart attack, surgery, car accident). Other traumatic events that go on in a community are family violence, community crises, fires, natural disasters, and military action (war trauma for returning military personnel).

If one of your specialties is trauma recovery, create a brochure on this topic that you can provide to the following potential referral sources. These are agencies and professionals that have first contact with individuals who have been traumatized:

- Fire departments
- Police
- Hospitals
- Ambulance companies
- Car insurance companies
- Personal injury attorneys
- Local emergency officials
- Chiropractors
- Auto body repair shops

To help your referral sources understand and know how and when to make a referral, offer free or low-fee psychoeducational workshops in your office, on site, or at a community center. You could offer psychoeducational workshops such as "Help for Victims of Violence" or "Feeling Safe in a Dangerous World."

Certification. You can become certified in this specialty by the International Critical Incident Stress Foundation in Ellicott City, Maryland, contact: (410)750-9600. They publish the *Journal of Emergency Medical Services*, which is full of good information.

Grief relief workshops can be offered and referrals received from clergy, physicians, nursing homes, hospices, funeral directors, and flower shop owners.

Grief Work

Community members also regularly lose important people, pets, and things in their lives. Grief relief workshops can be offered and referrals received from clergy, physicians, nursing homes, hospices, funeral directors,

The Alpha Centre

"A Safe Place To Talk"

Community Informational Series

Pet Loss & Grief

Office Location
6 Pleasant Street #214, Malden MA 02148
Communication Information
Mailing Address - PO Box 350 Melrose MA 02176
Voice Mail 781 662 6026 • FAX 781 662 8575
E Mail llawless@shore.net

Good-by Merlin

Loosing a pet can be a devastating experience, and a confusing one. You may ask questions like: "Why do I feel so upset about loosing my kitty?" "Why don't others understand how badly I feel? " What can I do to feel better?" It was only after the loss of Merlin, a cat I had owned for 15 years that I came to explore and understand what a painful and confusing experience pet loss can be.

Merlin, gave me what I, and many others, long for, unconditional love. Even though I have a loving family, all my adult relationships contain some type of condition. To my daughter I must remain in the role of mother, even though we expand the definition of mother as we both age. To my husband I am his life partner, and there are responsibilities I willingly assume. For my pussycat, the primary responsibility was to feed him and keep his litter box clean, and even that could be stretched. Merlin was at the door when I returned home, grumpy, from a long day's work. He happily jumped into my lap when I plopped down on the couch unable to talk without snapping to other's requests. When I was sick he slept beside me. When we moved he stayed near me as I readjusted to a new neighborhood. Merlin listened to my up and down times with the same nudge of my hand and a quick roll over to have his belly scratched. I still miss him dearly. I did not realize how devastated I would be when he died, after a long, costly bout with cancer. I am a trained mental health professional and did not realize how seriously depressed I was over his loss. "I can't feel this bad over a cat." "No one will understand." It wasn't until I looked at a video my husband had taken of our vacation right after Merlin passed that I realized that I was clinically depressed, over a cat. I had lost cats before, but Merlin was special. I was shocked to find how intense my grief was. Merlin held a very unique and special place in my heart, that no other pet, or person, had ever filled.

Luckily, other pet lovers allowed me to give myself permission to experience the depth of my grief. I was allowed time to feel numb after I had him put down because he was in such misery. I spent days struggling over the question, was I helping him by putting him to sleep, or myself? When he could no longer eat or walk to his litter box I knew it was time for him to die with some dignity. Then, after his death, I grew irritable with life. I cried for no reason, deeply and desperately. I felt hopeless, that I would never find anyone to take Merlin's place. It took months for me to return to "normal."

Eventually, two years later, I was asked to give a home to a rescue cat, Lilly, who had been abandoned in a woodpile and had lost an eye. She was tiny and had been very mistreated. She was frightened, dehydrated and near death after the removal of an infected eye. We checked each other out cautiously and found we could live with each other. I don't know who was getting cared for the most. Lilly physically and emotionally, or me emotionally. I was taking a great risk, opening my heart to another kitty.

Looking back I realize that people need help with many decisions and reactions to the death of a pet:

- When is it time to say goodbye and how will you arrange it?
- Putting the loss into some kind of context to match the depth of emotion that emerges.
- Sorting out the grief for the current loss from unresolved grief over other losses.
- Feeling guilty about grieving over the loss of a mere pet.
- Talking to children about pet loss.
- Deciding what to do with your pet's remains.
- How to memorialize your pet.
- If and when to bring another pet into your life.

Some recommendations I now make are:

- Take good care of yourself when you loose a pet. Don't minimize your feelings, they are true and important.
- Reach out and don't go it alone. Talk with people who understand and offer support.
- Get plenty of rest and watch what you eat. Food will not replace your pet. Eat nutritiously and beware of using substances to numb the pain.
- Use a journal to write letters to your pet. Express your feelings and tell them all the things you hope they will understand.
- Take one day at a time and know this too will pass.

If you find you need some help to get over the loss of a beloved pet, and have exhausted your own resources, call the Alpha Centre for an evaluation of your situation. It could be you are progressing naturally through grief. It may also be that you are stuck and need some help to move on. Take the simple assessment that follows to determine if your grief is more than normal grieving.

Simple Self Assessment

- I am eating more or less than usual.
- I am loosing days at work.
- I am using alcohol or other substances to numb the pain.
- My deep emotions have been going on for over three months.
- I don't have anyone to talk to about my feelings.
- I feel hopeless and want to end things.

The Alpha Centre offers counseling and consultation for "animal families." We address issues such as:

- Pet loss
- Pet abuse
- Deciding to own a pet
- Family problems that revolve around a pet
- Choosing a pet as a companion
- Problem pet behaviors

We have a network of animal specialists that we refer to and consult when necessary. The licensed mental health professionals at the Alpha Centre are family and relationship specialists. Please call for more information to make an appointment.

Call 781.322.3051

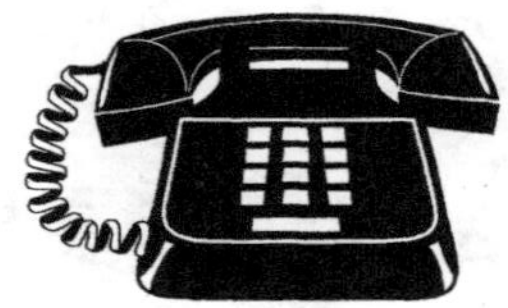

FIGURE 9.2 Pet Loss Informational Brochure

and flower shop owners. A specialty that is often overlooked in the area of grief is recovery from the loss of a pet. Resources include:

- Pet Loss Support Hotline at UC California at Davis www.vetnet.ucdavis.edu/petloss/index.htm
- The Pet Loss Support Hotline: (530) 752-4200; Hotline University of Florida (352) 392-4700.
- Virtual Pet Cemetery (www.lavamind.com/pet_ord3.html) where you can send a goodbye letter. They do ask for a donation.

The pet loss informational brochure in Figure 9.2 on pages 302–303 can be left in veterinarian offices, grooming waiting rooms, and kennels.

Refer to the resources at the end of this chapter for books on this topic.

A National Mental Health Association (NMHA) Chapter

Clifford Beers, a former psychiatric patient, started the NMHA in 1909. He started the organization to "expose and correct the injustices he observed and experienced during his hospitalizations for Bipolar Disorder." If there is already an NMHA chapter in your area, you can use their well-prepared mental health informational pamphlets, on which they will print your name and logo. They are very high quality. Topics include:

- Mental illness in the family.
- Anxiety disorders.
- Bipolar disorders.
- Overcoming depression.
- Several pamphlets for children and teens.

If there is not a chapter in your region, NMHA will send you an affiliate development guidebook that takes you step-by-step through developing a chapter. As you set up a chapter, you will learn organization, marketing, market research, fund raising, grant writing, and more. You will have a good way to meet local citizens, school administrators, and local agencies. Yes, it is a lot of work and so are other marketing programs. The association can be reached at (800) 969-NMHA and their web site at www.nmha.org. They have a fax on demand number (888) 836-6070.

More Topics and Approaches. Community related topics are endless; a few more to get you thinking are:

- *Helping Someone with Mental Illness* (Carter, 1998).
- Managing chronic disease (e.g., diabetes, cancer, HIV).
- Pain control.
- Geropsychiatric services.
- Anger management.

Community Theater

You might sponsor a community theater event that focuses on mental health or illness. It can be a very powerful and provocative tool to connect and relate to the community. Ideally, you would create a discussion group after watching a play. We recently attended a theater production of Shakespeare's *Hamlet.* After the performance, a psychologist from the Boston Psychoanalytic Institute sat with those who elected to remain and discussed the psychological issues woven throughout the play. We were amazed to find that at least a third of the audience remained for the discussion. You can also use this model with local theater pieces that touch on mental health issues. The Bureau for At-Risk Youth publishes a specialized catalog for videos that can be used with children and their parents. Refer to the Resources section for contact information.

Financially Accessible Practitioners

The Gap Network is a group of mental health professionals that work cooperatively to promote services that are affordable and an alternative to managed care. If you are interested in this concept, they can be reached at (617) 244-5542.

Public Relations

Marketing to the community is better framed as public relations. The objective of public relations is to develop your relationship with your target

The objective of public relations is to develop your relationship with your target market.

market. Before you begin your outreach, your market position must be clear. Communicate regularly with your niche market through media releases and other mediums, such as radio, television and community events. It is essential that the public have a positive view of all your outreach efforts. When a negative piece goes out, use your crisis intervention skills to reframe and repair the damage.

The media are present-moment focused. They face deadlines on a daily basis, in television on a minute-to-minute basis. Time and exposure lost can never be retrieved. The best way to deal with media staff is to help them meet their deadlines with quality information that benefits their genre. The best preparation for working with the media is to do your homework and be prepared to bend to their time deadlines. If they say they need an article or interview in 24 hours, don't take 25.

Speak their language. Learn about journalistic writing. The standard process-oriented dialogue you have with your peers is not going to cut it with the media. They want "talking points" and "sound bites." Have your facts arranged in a hierarchy. The most important points come first. Have fill-in information in case they need to expand an article or the interviewee preceding you does not show. When they view you as a competent resource, they will return to you over and over again. Reference books that help you identify media staff are the *Editor and Publisher International Yearbook* and *Bacon's Publicity Checker.*

Every media release needs to sing the same song. You can ensure this by creating a basic business statement as described in earlier chapters. This statement includes your mission and purpose, goals, primary services and products you are offering, their benefits, and your unique selling principle. Out of this will come a brief key message (e.g., "We offer quality mental health services, to create and support mental/emotional health, which in turn, we hope, produces a healthy, caring community"). Memorize this key message and include it in all your presentations. The next section describes a longer marketing script, which you might use at any networking event.

Marketing Script

Use the following formula to develop your script. This formula ensures an *authentic marketing* message. Before you complete the formula, decide to whom you are presenting this message, and what you are offering them. Once you are clear about your target audience, tell them:

- *Who You Are.* This needs to be information about who you are in relation to the service/product you are offering. Use language they understand. For example, "I am Linda Lawless, I'm a counselor in private practice in Malden, Massachusetts."
- *What You Do.* What you do needs to be as concrete as possible. If you offer services, be very clear about what they are: "I counsel women who have problems bingeing on food."
- *Why You Do It.* This builds a link between your services and you. It builds trust and offers a context for the person you are communicating with: "I have found that women who binge are often using the food as a distraction to feelings they find uncomfortable. When they begin to deal with these feelings, they discover a new sense of personal power and control over their lives. I get a great deal of satisfaction out of my work when my clients replace unhealthy habits with ones that help them grow and change. When they get stronger, they are better equipped to help their families and friends grow and change."
- *Why They Might Be Interested in What You Do.* This helps the person receiving the message position the information in their context: "Many women feel out of control over their eating habits and are afraid to ask for help. Finding the right kind of help can be a wonderful gift. I find as individuals get healthier, they help create healthier families and communities, which is a win-win for us all."
- *If They Are Interested, How People Can Reach You.* Tell them how people can begin to work with you. This is the time to hand them your business card and invite them to events at your office or offer the use of your resource center. Remember to specify what services are free and what an introductory consultation costs. "Anyone can come in and use our mental wellness resource center for free. If they are interested in exploring other services, we offer an introductory consultation for $25. We identify what services may be helpful for them and offer referrals to any services we do not offer. Just call me at (123) 456-7891 anytime. If I'm not available, our answering system gives directions on how to arrange a telephone appointment call-back."

With this script under your belt you are ready to expand into a larger public relations plan.

Working with the Media

Build your professional credibility and market acceptance.

Backgrounder. The first step in preparing a good public relations plan is to develop a relationship with media staff. Build your professional credibility and market acceptance. When you are beginning your public coming-out, do your homework and create a company background piece, which includes your history, services and specialties, and the market you work with. This creates a context for who you are and your position in the marketplace.

Press Kit. Putting together a press kit will help you get the big picture on You Inc. Your press kit does not need to be extra slick, but it must be accurate. Your kit can include:

- *Company Backgrounder.* This should describe how you started in the field, how you have grown, and the important experiences that shaped your growth and future direction. It can be in a written, audio, or video format. If you move to a video or multimedia presentation, use a professional media producer.
- *Tip Sheet.* Provide producers and editors with topic ideas and show the breadth of your expertise. Use your specialties as issue ideas (e.g., stress—family stress, stress in the workplace, medical complications due to stress). Link your informational pieces to these topics.
- *Public Service Announcements.* These are 10- to 60-second "spots" that can be used on radio and television. They provide a short message and can be in written, audio, or video format. If you use a video format, have it professionally produced.
- *Question Sheets.* Provide questions an interviewer can use to develop dialogue. Stay as clear of psychological jargon as you can.
- *Service and Product Descriptions.*
- *Copies of Your Newsletter and Brochures.*
- *One Sheets* on published books you have authored.
- *Press Releases* about awards you have received.
- *Newspaper or Periodic Publication Articles* in which you were quoted or highlighted.
- *Media Releases* about your workshops or presentations.

- *Thank-You Letters* from successful presentations.
- *Your Business Card.*
- A *Rolodex Card* for their file.
- A *Stress Card* imprinted with your name.

And whatever else you believe provides information about your business. Put all this information in a nice folder and give one to every media person you approach.

Outreach Letters. Create attention-grabbing letters to gain business media staff's attention. Then give them the information they need about your services and products in your press kit. After they have received your materials, call them and begin to develop the relationship. Maybe you want them to cover one of your community events. Tell them what your goals are and what you would like them to do. Ask them about their needs and interests and see if there is a win-win match. If there isn't one today, there may be one in the future. Continue to stay in touch, sending information about your new services and products, always asking them what they need from you. There are a few good ideas to follow in an outreach letter (Figure 9.3).

Telephone Pitch. Making telephone calls, especially to someone you do not know can be terrifying. A follow-up call to a mailing is a little easier. You can call simply to ask whether they have received your press kit and press release. Introduce yourself and your company and present your key message. Explain why you are calling and what you want. Give the media person a reason to continue to talk to you. Make sure you have done your homework about what you are offering to readers, listeners, or viewers. Ask the media person if this information is timely and, if not, what is needed. Find out what is on the reporter's agenda, and address those informational needs.

Give the media person a reason to continue to talk to you.

Press Releases. Your press release tells it all. Provide the following information:

- What are your services or products and why are they timely?
- How do consumers benefit from your services and products?
- What will it cost them?

Alpha Centre

6 Pleasant Street   Suite 214   Malden MA 02148   781-322-3051

Our mission is to be a professional resource in support of the health and well-being of

- The whole person
- Families
- Businesses, institutions, and
- Municipalities

in the service of creating caring community

Our services include psychoeducational workshops on:

EATING DISORDERS

HOW TO CHOOSE THE RIGHT THERAPIST

SELF-ESTEEM AND HEALTH

PARENTING TRAINING

COMMUNICATION SKILLS AND CONFLICT MANAGE-MENT

STRESS MANAGEMENT

MEDIATION

BEING A SUCCESSFUL SINGLE

SURVIVING AND THRIVING AS A STEP-FAMILY

FAMILY MEETINGS

MENTAL ILLNESS WHAT IS IT?

SUCCESSFUL AGING

SUCCESSFUL LIFESTYLE CHANGE

Family wellness supports a healthy community! (This is a headline that grabs the readers attention and leads them to read the letter)

Dear Malden Business Owner, (traditional salutation that specifies who they are.)

When your employees have family crises, they aren't able to concentrate on their job, and this affects your bottom line. Preventing a personal crisis can help you as well as your employee. *(Start with something that they will be interested in. What's in it for the reader to continue?)*

To protect your employees children the Alpha Centre is hosting Project KidCare. This program was created by the Polaroid Corporation and the National Center for Missing and Exploited Children and is being hosted at the Alpha Centre as a community service. We invite you and your employees to stop by with their families to have a free picture taken of the child/ren. Each photo is placed in a book with the child's vital information. This book is kept by the parents in a safe place, in case the child is ever found missing. It can be used by the Police and other agencies that help search for the child.

We expect to receive many calls to reserve photo opportunities. *(Create some urgency to contacting you.)* Please have one of your staff call the Alpha Centre to reserve times specifically for your employees. *(Tell them exactly what you want them to do.)*

Sincerely,

P.S. Don't be the only employer that didn't take advantage of a free employee benefit. Call today to reserve space.

FIGURE 9.3 Community Outreach Letter

- How do they access your services and how will they use them to their benefit?

Offer a quote from yourself about the needfulness of the service or product and your professional perspective on it. Position yourself in relation to the larger market or profession, so they have a context to understand what you are presenting to them. Also inform them about other alternatives and accessible community resources. To get your press release to the public:

- Know what the deadlines are. Make yourself user friendly by getting your information to the right person in a timely manner. Events that are closest to the publication date usually receive the highest priority.
- All your release information needs to be typed or computer generated, not handwritten. Don't use all capital letters; they are boring to the eye.
- Use the inverted-pyramid style of writing. You put the most important information first. Who you are, what you are informing people about, where and when it is happening. If you are announcing an event, the information should all be in the first paragraph.

It is unlikely that your information will be printed verbatim. If you want a photographer to attend your event, give them plenty of notice. You can send your own photograph with your press release. We recommend using a professionally created photograph. If you do not have one, you can contact their professional associations:

- Advertising Photographers of America (310) 201-0781.
- American Society of Media Photographers (609) 799-8300.
- Professional Photographers of America (404) 522-8600.

Look for credentials and experience in publicity or fashion photography. Before your photo event, see a makeup specialist who deals with preparing models for photographs. If you don't know such a specialist, once you identify a good media photographer, ask for a referral to a makeup/hair expert. When you choose a high quality photograph to send, include a photocopy that indicates the individual/s correct name and their position in the photo.

Press Release Worksheet. Your services deserve press coverage, and many media staff are under deadline pressure. Press releases that are not easy to read and don't contain the information needed disappear in the round file. The following outline will help you create your own piece:

- The business name and the services provided.
- What is being announced.
- When it is happening or is available.
- What you want people to do or understand.
- Your key message which can include:
  - What the services do in terms of benefits.
  - Why these benefits are necessary and timely.
  - How the services are different from services that others provide.
  - What kinds of people use these services.
  - The benefits they get out of using them.
  - Your businesses position message for the marketplace.
  - When these services are not helpful.
  - Alternatives to these services.
  - Community resources for these problems.
  - A quote from you about the services.
  - Supporting credentials and awards.
  - More detailed contact information.

Obtain permission to reprint the article, radio presentation, or video event in your other outreach activities, and to include it in your press kit.

After one of your press releases has been used, send a thank-you note to the media person who facilitated its publication. If the release is for an event, invite the media to attend, take pictures, and create a news story for the community. After the event or publication, obtain permission to reprint the article, radio presentation, or video event in your other outreach activities, and to include it in your press kit. After it is all over, arrange a press interview for other media people who might be interested. A sample press release and worksheet is shown in Figure 9.4.

For Immediate Release

Name of Organization

Address

Contact's Name

Contact's Telephone and Fax Number

Linda Lawless and Jean Wright of the Alpha Centre (who you are), are opening (what you are doing) their office doors on Wednesday, January 27 at 10 A.M. (when you are doing it) to the Malden community, and invite you to come by the office at 6 Pleasant Street, Suite 214 (where you are doing it), and join in their celebration (what you want them to do). The Alpha Centre's mission is to bring quality mental health resources to everyone in need and be an information resource to the community (your central message).

"Many people wonder what mental illness, mental wellness and a healthy family is. We help answer those questions, serve during a time of crisis, and facilitate greater understanding of mental wellness through our workshops and our free resource center," (quote) said (your name) Ms. Wright, who (primary qualification) is a Licensed Marriage and Family Therapist and clergywoman (secondary qualification).

The Alpha Centre's free resource center also provides referrals to other professionals when you are in need of services outside the scope of the Alpha Centre.

Ms. Wright does everything she can to help families raise healthy children. Through her work, she has been honored by the National Association of Family Advocates for helping single-parent women get back on their feet and move forward in rebuilding their lives (awards, qualifications, and positions held).

The Alpha Centre is open Monday through Friday from 10 A.M. to 8 P.M. (list hours) and can be reached by Telephone (781) 322-3051 or e-mail at Jean@thealphacentre.com (contact information).

FIGURE 9.4 Sample Press Release and Worksheet

Events, products, and services all can be the topic of a press release. The press release shown in Figure 9.5 is specifically service oriented.

Letters to the Editor. Here is another way to get in print for the cost of time. You have probably read an article in a newspaper or magazine that made you want to talk back. Do it in print. These letters are also subject to

For Immediate Release

Name of Organization

Address

Contact's Name

Contact's Telephone and Fax Number

The Alpha Centre (group name) announces The Family Wellness Game (service name).

Malden, MA (city, state), Wednesday January 27 (date) The Alpha Centre (group name) today announced its Family Wellness Games for the month of February (time period). The game experience costs $25 (price) and meets every Friday during the month of February (how often) from 10 A.M. to 7 P.M. (starting date, ending date, and times) at their offices at 6 Pleasant Street, Suite 214 (location).

They will demonstrate how the Family Wellness Game is played and schedule a free game rental for your family. The Family Wellness Game is an activity every family will enjoy and learn from (elaboration of offering).

Register by calling the Alpha Centre at (781) 322-3051 (contact information) and reserving a time for your demonstration (what you want them to do).

The Alpha Centre offers quality mental health services, to create and support mental/emotional health, which in turn, we hope, produces a healthy, caring community. Healthy families are a fundamental part of a healthy community (key and/or positioning statement).

FIGURE 9.5 Service Program Press Release Template

editing. When you send your letter, be sure to include your name, address, telephone number and any other verification information. Be as succinct as possible and use some personal taste. These letters should be typed and double-spaced. Find out what the deadline is for the publication, and the name of the person who edits this section of the publication.

Public Speaking

Public speaking is the best community marketing approach we know of for mental health counselors. It allows potential consumers and referral agents to see and hear you and begin to trust your expertise. There are many resources to help you develop speaking skills. If you are new to public speaking, try Toastmasters. They offer an excellent training program and are national. You can locate a group near you by calling Toastmasters at (714) 858-8255 and asking for a print-out of meetings in your area. When you have developed basic speaking skills, the place to learn the business of speaking is the National Speakers Association. They can be reached at (602) 698-2552. A great speaker resource is the Therapist Presentation Kit. This kit was prepared by Laurie Grand and includes 17 prepared presentations including overheads, script, and handouts. Topics include Understanding Depression, Single Parent Survival Skills, Understanding Anger, and more. The kit includes presentation pointers and Tips for Marketing Your Practice. There are also presentations on marriage that include:

When you have developed basic speaking skills, the place to learn the business of speaking is the National Speakers Association.

- Before the Wedding.
- How to Build a Good Marriage.
- The Marriage Check-Up.
- Recovering from Infidelity.

The kit can be purchased from Laurie Grand, M.S. by calling (847) 304-0385, or you can visit her web site at www.free-agent-therapist.com.

Before you rule out public speaking because it terrifies you, remember that you are public speaking every time you tell someone about who you are and what you do. There are many forums for public speaking:

- Adult education classes.
- Academic classes.

For each public presentation, you need to have a goal in mind.

- Lunchtime presentations to service organizations.
- Keynote speeches to your professional association.
- Psychoeducation presentations to the community.
- Partnering with another professional and presenting at their workshop.
- Being on a panel of experts.

The art of public speaking is a learned skill that you combine with your presentation style. For each public presentation, you need to have a goal in mind. When you introduce yourself at a networking event or present a daylong workshop, have an outcome in mind. At the networking event, it could be to hand out at least 25 cards. At the workshop, it could be to gain three new consultation visits. The fundamental model for a speech is:

- *Opening*. Who you are and what you do and why you do it.
- *Point 1*. The most basic point about the topic you are addressing.
- *Support* for this point. Includes why the listeners might be interested in your topic.
- *Point 2* about this topic.
- *Point 3* about this topic. Why they might be interested in working with you.
- *Conclusion*. What you want them to do to support your goal for this presentation and how they can reach you if they want to.

There are many good books on public speaking. A useful one that was written by a mental health professional is *Marketing with Speeches and Seminars*, by Miriam Ottee (1998).

Workshops and Seminars

Workshops and seminars are in the genre of public speaking and are more highly structured. When you present a training workshop on a topic, you are positioning yourself as an expert in the field. This more structured model is often easier for a mental health professional to accomplish when they are beginning to go public. The process of presenting successful workshops is to first identify your target market, select a topic they would be interested in, design your workshop, market and present it. All along the way, there are resources to help you. To identify a topic for a niche market go to the library or the Internet and read the information and publications this population reads. You will see advertisements for workshops in their periodicals and articles about areas of interest. The focus group is also a good market research tool for this project. You need to differentiate between perceived versus actual needs. You may know a niche market needs some skills but they may not recognize that need. The ideal solution is a real need that your market perceives as a need. The successful workshop will also be designed to speak the language of the target audience. A workshop on anxiety disorders will be different for parents of children with ADHD than it will be for your colleagues.

To identify a topic for a niche market go to the library or the Internet and read the information and publications this population read.

Your workshop content needs to include the information your audience wants and needs, new skills they can apply, and attitudes that support referrals. Your workshop objectives need to be concrete and measurable. The flow of the workshop agenda should be designed to meet the educational needs of your audience. If you are speaking to adults, use an adult educational model that includes lecture and individual or group experiential exercises. There are many tools to keep attendees involved (e.g., games, videos, structured tasks, group interaction).

The field of workshops, seminars, and training is enormous with many resources including training and development associations, books, and tools. Valuable publications are:

Friedman, R.J., & Altman, P. (1997). *How to design, develop, and market healthcare seminars.* (Sarasota, FL: Professional Resource Press).

Greenbaum, I.L. (1993). *The handbook for focus group research.* (New York: Lexington Books).

Jolles, R.L. (1993). *How to run seminars and workshops.* (New York: John Wiley & Sons).

Shenson, H.L. (1990). *How to develop and promote successful seminars and workshops.* (New York: John Wiley & Sons).

Newspapers, Television, and Radio

Television and radio outreach may seem out of your reach or expertise but both can be accessible and a valuable piece of your marketing mix.

Advertising in these media is expensive, but there are other ways. For example, our nonprofit education corporation, Metro-Boston Professional Counseling Network, provided a cable network weekly program on mental health issues. The cable station provided the training we needed to produce and present our call-in program, and in the process we all learned new personal presentation techniques as well as a great deal about the community at large.

To bring your services and products to the media's attention to gain free exposure, you need to know the key players.

To bring your services and products to the media's attention to gain free exposure, you need to know the key players. In the world of broadcast, identify the program director, producer, public affairs director, and reporters for news programs. When approaching newspapers, learn the names of the managing editor, city editor, editor, and reporters. All this information is available through a simple phone call. Armed with these names, you can direct your press releases and ideas for programming to the right person.

Begin with your local community. When you feel comfortable and in some kind of control of your media coverage, expand to regional and national.

Television. If you are entering the television media, you can begin with a local cable offering and advance to a full-blown program. A finished program requires scripting for everything that is seen and heard. It will include script for the "talent" and announcer, music, background noise, still pictures, animation, set design, staging, and audience participation. Remember to dress for television. Consult your producer about what to wear for best visual impact.

Television or Radio. If you choose to be interviewed on a topic, remember to:

- Know your message and have backup statements with facts and figures.
- Approach the topic from the audience's and reporter's perspective. Do your research on public perspective and educate the interviewer about your perspective.
- Think in small "sound bites." Consumers are used to short messages. Don't ramble on about a process. Provide facts and short informational statements.

- Stay in control. If you are thrown off, come back to center, and if you need to ask what you were talking about before you were distracted, ask, rather than mumble on.
- Be yourself. Everyone can see through a false presentation.
- Connect with the interviewer. This will facilitate connecting with your audience.
- Project energy, optimism, and enthusiasm.

Organization:

Alpha Centre

6 Pleasant Street #214

Malden MA 02148

Contact Person:

Linda Lawless & Co. Telephone (781) 322-3051

For Immediate Release: Start Date 12/1/98

Words = 115
Time 30 Seconds

METIS—A Holiday Support Group

During the holiday season are you constantly fighting the diet dragon? Do you find yourself thinking about food throughout the day? Have holiday gatherings become an uncomfortable time of fighting temptation?

Make this the year you give yourself the priceless gift of peace of mind.

Rid yourself of the constant torment of thinking about food, struggling with food choices, and not enjoying holiday events.

The Alpha Centre in Malden is offering a free gift to the community. It is a support group for anyone who wants help to be free of unhealthy food thinking, and food choice struggles. Call the Alpha Centre at (781) 322-3051 for the time and place of these groups.

Figure 9.6 Media Release

Radio. Many radio stations present one-minute community service announcements. You have the best chance for a spot if you are a not-for-profit corporation, but if you are offering a free public service, you have a shot at it. Figure 9.6 on page 319 provides a sample 30-second announcement about a free support group.

When you are ready for national exposure, we recommend contacting *Radio-TV Interview Report.* It is a magazine that is sent out to over 4,000 radio and television talk show producers. To get started, you choose the issues you want to advertise in (they publish biweekly) and send a copy of your press materials, a photo, and any publications you have that support your expertise. Contact the magazine and ask for an information packet. They can be reached at (800) 989-1400.

Summary

Marketing to your community will open doors you never knew existed. Done right, your return on investment will exceed your expenses. Ideally, cross-fertilization occurs, enriching you and those you connect with. Public relations is the nature of the relationship you create. The media is the voice of your message.

Resources

Calendars of Events

"Health Observances and Recognition Day Calendar," contact: Society for Healthcare Strategy and Market Development (800) 242-2626.

Chase's Calendar of Events—The Day-to-Day Directory to Special Days, Weeks, and Months (312) 540-4500.

Community

City Link www.banzai.neosoft.com/citylink/ma.html

City Net www.city.net/countries/united_states/massachusetts/

National Issues Forums (800)433-7834

Yahoo! Government www.yahoo.com/Government/

Photographers

Advertising Photographers of America—(310) 201-0781

American Society of Media Photographers—(609) 799-8300

Professional Photographers of America—(404) 522-8600

Professional Associations

Association for the Advancement of Applied Sports Psychology—www.aasponline.org

The International Critical Incident Stress Foundation—www.icisf.org

Public Speaking

Grand. L., Free Agent Therapist
1250 West Grove Avenue, Suite 200
Barrington, IL 60010
(847) 304-8385

National Speakers Association
1500 South Priest Drive
Tempe, AZ 85281
(602) 968-2552
www.nsaspeaker.org

ToastMasters
P.O. Box 9052
Mission Viejo, CA 92690
(949) 858-8255

Theater Productions

Ki Theatre—(540) 987-3164 and www.pobox.com/-ki.theatre

The Bureau for At-Risk Youth; Promoting Growth Through Knowledge
135 Dupont Street, P.O. Box 760
Plainview, NY 11803-0760
(800) 99-YOUTH

Recommended Reading

The Journal of Applied Sport Psychology (800)627-0629

The Group Circle: The Newsletter of the American Group Psychotherapy Association. (1999, February/March).

The Inner Edge: A Resource for Enlightened Business Practice (800)899-1712

Brandt, B. (1995). *Whole life economics.* New York: New Society.

Carter, R. (1998). *Helping someone with mental illness: A compassionate guide for family, friends, and caregivers.* New York: Random House.

Friedman, R.J., & Altman, P. (1997). *How to design, develop, and market healthcare seminars.* (Sarasota, FL: Professional Resource Press).

Greenbaum, I.L. (1993). *The handbook for focus group research.* (New York: Lexington Books).

Hopkins, M. (1998, August/September). In a "healthy city," no one is superfluous. *The Inner Edge,* 1.

Jolles, R.L. (1993). *How to run seminars and workshops.* (New York: John Wiley & Sons).

Lawless, L. (1997). *Therapy Inc.* New York: Wiley.

Mahoney, D., & Restak, R. (1998). *The longevity strategy: How to live to 100 using the brain-body connection.* New York: Wiley.

Otte, M. (1998). *Marketing with speeches and seminars.* Seattle, WA: Zest Press.

Quackenbush, J., & Graveline, D. (1985). *When your pet dies: How to cope with your feelings.* New York: Simon & Schuster.

Shenson, H.L. (1990). *How to develop and promote successful seminars and workshops.* (New York: John Wiley & Sons).

Stearns, A.K. (1984). *Living through personal crisis.* New York: Ballantine Books.

Williams, R. (1994). *The non-designer's design book: Design and typographic principles for the visual novice.* Berkeley, CA: PeachPit Press.

Williams, R. (1996). *Beyond the MAC is not a typewriter.* Berkeley, CA: PeachPit Press.

Williams, T.A. (1997). *Kitchen-table publisher.* Coral Springs, FL: Venture Press.

Closing Summary

You help create a community standard of quality mental healthcare, which begins with honoring your professional life. The most important thing you can do is commit to your responsibility for the success of your professional practice.

The information, worksheets, and resources in this book provide you with a foundation to build success. Success is not a goal; it is a process in the dynamic mental healthcare marketplace. As this book was being printed, more resources and ideas were being generated.

This evolving context is the one in which you will grow and mature as a mental health professional. Please share your creativity and insights into how to use this book with colleagues in your community. Getting referrals can be either an individual or a group endeavor. This book facilitates both approaches. Please share your experiences of using this material with us; we welcome your feedback. E-mail us at Jean or Linda at thealphacentre.com.

We are co-responsible for the future of the mental healthcare profession. One success contributes to the success of all. We wish you the best in your professional success.

Index

www.ingramcontent.com/pod-product-compliance
Lightning Source LLC
LaVergne TN
LVHW060559240826
846221LV00003B/24